ROSS LABORATORIES

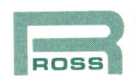

Y0-CLE-160

625 CLEVELAND AVENUE/COLUMBUS, OHIO 43215
(614) 624-7677
A DIVISION OF ABBOTT LABORATORIES, USA

Dear Doctor:

We are pleased to present the Report of the 102nd Ross Conference on Pediatric Research, **Hearing Loss in Childhood: A Primer.**

We think you will find this "primer" to be a comprehensive and valuable educational tool and reference source for pediatric and family practice professionals. Included are discussions of sensorineural and conductive hearing loss, testing/screening methods, developmental and educational effects, case management, and patient advocacy.

These are followed by two reference segments: **Appendix A** contains the Joint Committee on Infant Hearing 1990 Position Statement, to help identify infants at risk for hearing impairment and provide appropriate intervention and follow-up. **Appendix B** is a directory of individuals and agencies that provide information and services for patients, parents, and physicians.

We thank the expert participants whose knowledge we share with the pediatric community in this report.

Sincerely,

Clinton A. Johnson
Director
Professional Services

Henry S. Sauls, MD, FAAP
Vice President
Medical Affairs

Hearing Loss in Childhood: A Primer

Report of the 102nd Ross Conference on Pediatric Research
Published by Ross Laboratories
Columbus, Ohio 43216

ROSS CONFERENCES
on Pediatric Research

The 102nd Ross Conference on Pediatric Research was held in Tucson, Arizona, March 24-27, 1991. This Conference was one of a series designed to present findings from recent research on subjects pertaining to pediatrics and to stimulate further research by the exchange of information.

Director, Professional Services	Clinton A. Johnson Ross Laboratories
Associate Director, Professional Services	Jeffrey B. Head Ross Laboratories
Medical Editors	Roland D. Eavey, MD *Harvard Medical School* Jerome O. Klein, MD *Boston University School of Medicine*
Editorial Services Manager	Dorothy E. Redfern Ross Laboratories
Editorial Assistant	Oather J. Talley II Ross Laboratories
Vice President, Medical Affairs	Henry S. Sauls, MD, FAAP Ross Laboratories

©1992 Ross Laboratories　　　　　　　　　　M5789/March 1992
Printed in USA
Library of Congress Catalog Card No. 91-68122
Quotation permitted if source acknowledged. Preferred form: Author and title, in Eavey RD, Klein JO (eds): *Hearing Loss in Childhood: A Primer*, Report of the 102nd Ross Conference on Pediatric Research. Columbus, Ohio: Ross Laboratories, 1992, p 00.

Ross Laboratories is privileged to be associated with the production and provision of this information to members of the medical profession. Compilation and publication of this information constitute neither approval nor endorsement by Ross Laboratories or Abbott Laboratories of the opinions, inferences, findings, or conclusions stated or implied by the authors in the presentations.

Ross Laboratories
Columbus, Ohio 43216
Division of Abbott Laboratories, USA

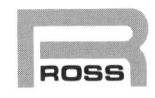

Hearing Loss in Childhood: A Primer

Chairpersons

Roland D. Eavey, MD
    Director
ENT Pediatric Services
Massachusetts Eye and Ear Infirmary
Assistant Professor of Otology and Laryngology
Harvard Medical School
Boston, Massachusetts

Jerome O. Klein, MD
    Director
Division of Pediatric Infectious Diseases
Boston City Hospital
Professor of Pediatrics
Boston University School of Medicine
Boston, Massachusetts

Participants

Fred H. Bess, PhD
    Chief Executive Officer
Bill Wilkerson Center
Professor and Director
Division of Hearing and Speech Sciences
Vanderbilt University School of Medicine
Nashville, Tennessee

Patrick E. Brookhouser, MD
    Director
Boys Town National Research Hospital
Omaha, Nebraska

Cynthia Chase, PhD
    Assistant Professor of Psychiatry
and Pediatrics
Boston University School of Medicine
Neuropsychology Service
Boston City Hospital
Boston, Massachusetts

Jerome T. Combs, MD, FAAP
    Primary Care Pediatrician
Wallingford, Connecticut

Michael J. Cunningham, MD, FAAP — *Assistant Professor of Otology and Laryngology Harvard Medical School Assistant Surgeon Department of Otolaryngology Massachusetts Eye and Ear Infirmary Boston, Massachusetts*

Julia M. Davis, PhD — *Dean College of Liberal Arts University of Minnesota Minneapolis, Minnesota*

Peter A. de Villiers, PhD — *Professor of Psychology Smith College Northampton, Massachusetts*

Philip R. Dodge, MD — *Professor of Pediatrics and Neurology Acting Director Division of Pediatric Neurology Washington University School of Medicine St Louis, Missouri*

Lynne V. Feagans, PhD — *Professor of Human Development and Family Studies Pennsylvania State University University Park, Pennsylvania*

Dennis Gjerdingen, MS — *President Clarke School for the Deaf/ Center for Oral Education Northampton, Massachusetts*

Kenneth M. Grundfast, MD, FACS, FAAP — *Professor of Pediatrics and Otolaryngology George Washington University School of Medicine Chairman, Department of Otolaryngology Children's National Medical Center Washington, DC*

Chris Halpin, PhD — *Clinical Associate Department of Audiology Massachusetts Eye and Ear Infirmary Instructor Department of Otology and Laryngology Harvard Medical School Boston, Massachusetts*

Paul E. Hammerschlag, MD — *Clinical Associate Professor of Otolaryngology*
New York University School of Medicine
New York, New York

Jo-Ann S. Harris, MD, FAAP — *Assistant Clinical Professor of Pediatrics*
Boston University School of Medicine
Boston, Massachusetts

Montgomery C. Hart, MD — *Medical Director*
Regional Perinatal Laboratory
Phoenix, Arizona

Barbara S. Herrmann, PhD — *Clinical Associate*
Audiology Department
Massachusetts Eye and Ear Infirmary
Boston, Massachusetts

M. Charles Liberman, PhD — *Associate Professor of Otology and Laryngology*
Harvard Medical School
and Massachusetts Eye and Ear Infirmary
Boston, Massachusetts

William M. Luxford, MD — *Associate*
House Ear Clinic
Los Angeles, California

Stephen I. Pelton, MD — *Professor of Pediatrics*
Boston University School of Medicine
Boston, Massachusetts

Robert J. Ruben, MD, FACS, FAAP — *Professor and Chairperson*
Department of Otolaryngology
Professor of Pediatrics
Albert Einstein College of Medicine
of Yeshiva University
and the Montefiore Medical Center
New York, New York

Sylvan E. Stool, MD — *Professor of Otolaryngology and Pediatrics*
University of Pittsburgh School of Medicine
Director of Education
Department of Pediatric Otolaryngology
Children's Hospital of Pittsburgh
Pittsburgh, Pennsylvania

Aaron Thornton, PhD *Assistant Professor of Otology and Laryngology Harvard Medical School Director of Audiology Massachusetts Eye and Ear Infirmary Boston, Massachusetts*

Bonnie P. Tucker, JD *Law Professor Arizona State University Tempe, Arizona Partner, Brown and Bain, PA Phoenix, Arizona*

Sumner J. Yaffe, MD *Director Center for Research for Mothers and Children National Institute of Child Health and Human Development National Institutes of Health Bethesda, Maryland*

Contents

Introduction and Purpose of Meeting
Roland D. Eavey, MD, and Jerome O. Klein, MD 1

Session I—Sensorineural Hearing Loss: Epidemiology, Etiology, and Pathogenesis

Sensorineural Hearing Loss in Newborn Infants
Michael J. Cunningham, MD 2

Genetic Deafness and Hearing Impairment in Childhood
Kenneth M. Grundfast, MD 9

Deafness in Children Related to Meningitis
Philip R. Dodge, MD 18

Ototoxicity
Jo-Ann S. Harris, MD 25

Loud Sound: Ear Damage, Hearing Loss, and Ear Protection
M. Charles Liberman, PhD 32

Session II—Conductive Hearing Loss: Epidemiology, Etiology, and Pathogenesis

Hearing Loss and Otitis Media:
Epidemiology, Etiology, and Pathogenesis
Jerome O. Klein, MD 41

Structural Reasons for Conductive Hearing Loss
Roland D. Eavey, MD 45

Session III—Hearing Testing

Audiometry Primer
Barbara S. Herrmann, PhD 55

Neonatal Screening
Aaron Thornton, PhD 61

Recognition of the Hearing-Impaired Patient in a
Primary-Care Pediatric Practice
Jerome T. Combs, MD 68

Screening School-Age Children for Auditory Function
Fred H. Bess, PhD 74

Session IV—Effects of Hearing Loss on Development

Speech and Language Development
Lynne V. Feagans, PhD 82

Hearing Loss and Development:
A Neuropsychologic Perspective
Cynthia Chase, PhD 88

Language and Speech as a Management Guide and Outcome Measure
Robert J. Ruben, MD 94

Session V—Management

Hearing Aids and Assistive Devices
Chris Halpin, PhD 103

Cochlear Implants in Children
William M. Luxford, MD 109

Intervention Strategies for the Child With Recurrent or Persistent Middle Ear Disease
Stephen I. Pelton, MD 115

Surgical Management To Decrease Hearing Impairment
Sylvan E. Stool, MD 120

Session VI—Educational Issues

Educational Implications of Deafness: Language and Literacy
Peter A. de Villiers, PhD 127

Evaluation, and Then What? What Pediatricians Should Know About Hearing Loss in Young Children
Dennis Gjerdingen, MS 135

Signing and Total Communication
Julia M. Davis, PhD 141

Session VII—Personal Experience

Reflections of a Hearing-Impaired Otologist
Paul E. Hammerschlag, MD 149

Session VIII—Advocacy

Guidelines for Physicians Who Treat
Hearing-Impaired Children
  Bonnie P. Tucker, JD 155

Appendix A:
**Joint Committee on Infant Hearing
1990 Position Statement** 162

Appendix B:
**Information Services
February 1991**
  Compiled by Bonnie P. Tucker, JD 166

Introduction and Purpose of Meeting

Roland D. Eavey, MD, and Jerome O. Klein, MD

Pediatricians are often requested to provide an opinion about a child's hearing. Yet many pediatric training programs do not provide extensive training for evaluation and management of hearing loss. One goal of this conference was to provide pediatricians and family physicians with insight into pertinent etiologies and pathogeneses of hearing loss to assist with patient management. Another goal was to provide information as to what type of care various specialists can provide to assist with patient referral. Finally, we hope that this publication will provide a valuable, practical reference to assist in the management of children with hearing impairment.

Session I—
Sensorineural Hearing Loss: Epidemiology, Etiology, and Pathogenesis

Sensorineural Hearing Loss in Newborn Infants
Michael J. Cunningham, MD

Points To Recall:
- *Specific clinical criteria (**Appendix A**) designate certain neonates to be at high risk for sensorineural hearing loss.*
- *All newborn infants who require NICU admission are at increased risk for sensorineural hearing loss.*

Consideration for Referral:
- *All children who fail a "high-risk" questionnaire regardless of gestational or postnatal age*

One of every 1,000 infants will be diagnosed by 3 years of age to have severely handicapping sensorineural hearing loss; an approximately equal number of children and young adults eventually will manifest severe to profound hearing loss of disabling proportions by age 19 years.[1] This prevalence of hearing impairment is increased significantly in selected neonatal populations. The focus of this paper is on those prenatal, intrapartum, and postnatal factors that identify a particular infant to be at "high risk" for sensorineural deafness.

Sensorineural hearing loss is classically differentiated as being either congenital or acquired in etiology. Congenital hearing loss is further subdivided into genetic and nongenetic categories (Table).

Approximately 50% of congenital sensorineural hearing loss is reportedly genetic.[2] The majority of affected children have hearing loss at birth; a smaller percentage will not develop their hearing impairment until later in childhood. The initial newborn assessment may provide clues to the underlying presence of a genetic hearing loss. In addition to a positive familial history, pertinent physical findings include evidence of cardiac, renal, pigmentary, craniofacial, and/or auricular malformation.

Nongenetic congenital deafness is attributable to intrapartum disease. The most commonly recognized type of nongenetic congenital deafness is due to maternal infection transmitted to the fetus transplacentally or through the cervix at the time of birth. The most common infectious agents are collectively grouped under the acronym *ToRCHeS* (*t*oxoplasmosis, *r*ubella, *c*ytomegalovirus, *h*erpes simplex, and *s*yphilis). Rubella and cytomegalovirus are of principal importance.

Table. Neonatal Sensorineural Hearing Loss: Potential Etiologies.

Congenital Disorders
  Genetic
    Present at birth
      Sensorineural hearing loss alone
      Syndromic sensorineural hearing loss
    Onset later in childhood
      Sensorineural hearing loss alone
      Syndromic sensorineural hearing loss
  Nongenetic
    Perinatal infection (ToRCHeS*)
    Maternal ototoxic medications/exposures
      Thalidomides
      Quinine
      Aminoglycosides
      Ethyl alcohol (?)
    Metabolic diseases
      Hypothyroidism
      Diabetes (?)
Perinatal Disorders
  Asphyxia/birth trauma
  Hyperbilirubinemia
  Necessity of NICU admission
  Neonatal meningitis/sepsis
  Noise trauma
  Ototoxic medications
  Prematurity/low birth weight

*Toxoplasmosis, rubella, cytomegalovirus, herpes simplex, syphilis

    Historically, rubella has been the most easily identifiable cause of congenital sensorineural deafness in children.[3] Sensorineural hearing loss occurs in approximately one third of rubella-infected infants. Although hearing loss can be an isolated finding, these neonates typically demonstrate other systemic manifestations of rubella infection, including physical and psychomotor retardation, thrombocytopenia with associated petechiae and purpura, hepatosplenomegaly, jaundice, cataracts and retinitis, congenital heart and renal defects, and both lower-limb and cranial deformities. The hearing loss in these children is often severe to profound, is generally asymmetric, and typically affects all frequencies evenly. The clinical suspicion of rubella can be confirmed serologically by documentation of rubella-specific IgM antibody, or persistence of neonatal rubella-specific IgG antibody following disappearance of maternal IgG levels, in the infant's blood. The aggressive vaccination of young women before childbearing age has significantly decreased the incidence of congenital rubella infection in developed countries.
    Cytomegalovirus (CMV) is currently established to be the most common intrapartum viral infection and is strongly suspected to be the most

common viral agent causing congenital sensorineural deafness in children.[3] Only 5% to 10% of CMV-infected neonates have clinically apparent disease; these children present with systemic manifestations very similar to those described for congenital rubella. Ninety to ninety-five percent of CMV-infected newborns have subclinical disease. In fact, up to 1% of all newborns reportedly demonstrate evidence of asymptomatic infection when saliva or urine is screened for the presence of CMV. Long-term follow-up of these subclinically CMV-infected children reveals that 7% to 13% of them eventually demonstrate sensorineural hearing loss.[4,5] This incidence of hearing impairment is far higher in children with symptomatic CMV infection, ranging from 20% to 65%.[4,5] CMV-induced hearing loss is typically severe to profound, asymmetric, and bilateral. There is currently no established means of preventing primary infection in at-risk mothers or effective therapy for treating congenitally infected infants. Several methods are available to screen for and detect congenital CMV infection, including culturing the virus from urine and documentation of CMV-specific IgM antibody in neonatal serum.

The sudden transition from womb to delivery room subjects the newborn infant to a variety of external factors and forced adaptations in the first hours, weeks, and months of life that appear to have particular significance in regard to future hearing status. This is particularly true of premature and severely ill term neonates who require intensive-care hospitalizations. The overall prevalence of moderate to profound hearing impairment among NICU survivors has been estimated at between 2% and 12%, or 20 to 100 times greater than that recorded in the infant population at large.[6-9] Neonates with birth weights < 1500 g appear to be at particular risk, with figures reported in the 9% to 17% range.[10,11] Severity of illness also appears to play a role, as even higher prevalences of sensorineural hearing loss have been documented in term infants with persistent fetal circulation[12] and in premature, low-birth-weight infants with neonatal-seizure histories.[10]

Much effort has been directed toward identifying individual variables associated with hearing impairment in the NICU population. One focus of attention has been noise trauma. Infant incubators produce continuous noise levels of between 50 and 86 dB hearing level (HL), with a low-frequency distribution maintained principally around 500 Hz.[13] Concern has been raised about the neonatal aspects of noise trauma for several reasons: Incubator-noise exposure is continuous, with no opportunity for recovery; animal studies suggest that infants may be more susceptible than adults to noise-induced hearing loss; and, perhaps most important, a synergistic effect may occur between noise trauma and other potential ototoxic stresses in the critically ill neonate. The potentiation of noise-induced hearing loss by aminoglycoside antibiotics has been established in animal studies for both kanamycin and neomycin.[14,15] Levels of continuous noise as low as 58 dB HL increased the risk of hearing loss from these agents. Based on this information, in 1974 the American Academy of Pediatrics Committee on Environmental Hazards recommended that all manufacturers reduce the noise of their incubator motors, preferably to below this level.[16] This recommendation, however, was made without clinical confirmation of an association between hearing loss and infants' length of stay in incubators when other NICU factors have been relatively controlled.[6]

Ototoxic medications in and of themselves have been investigated as a possible cause of sensorineural hearing loss in the neonatal population. Several studies attest to the low risk of ototoxicity following parenteral administration of aminoglycoside antibiotics in appropriate dosage to infants with normal renal function. Behavioral audiometric assessments of young children who had been treated with kanamycin or gentamicin as neonates have revealed no subsequent sensorineural hearing loss or vestibular dysfunction in these children compared to their non-antibiotic-treated peers; this has been true of both premature and full-term infant groups.[17,18] More recent work involving brain-stem auditory evoked-response (BAER) testing of infants after a minimum period of 5 weeks following cessation of aminoglycoside therapy reveals normal sensorineural hearing thresholds in all infant ears tested.[19] Such BAER testing is particularly noteworthy because the click stimulus that is used is especially sensitive in detecting hearing loss at the high-frequency 4000-Hz level, the frequency at which aminoglycoside-induced ototoxicity would initially be suspected to occur.

The role of asphyxia has been an additional focus of attention in terms of its contribution to sensorineural hearing impairment. An Apgar score of less than 4 at 10 minutes, laboratory evidence of acidosis (pH < 7.1), and clinical manifestations such as neonatal coma or seizure activity have been used as indicators of significant perinatal asphyxia. Proposed mechanisms of sensorineural hearing impairment include direct hypoxic injury to brain-stem auditory nuclei[20] and the extension of intracranial hemorrhage, a frequent clinical correlate of hypoxia and acidosis, into the inner ear labyrinth.[21] The increased prevalence of deafness among children with severe mental retardation and cerebral palsy has additionally been used as supportive evidence of the role of asphyxia in sensorineural hearing loss.[22] A definite correlation between Apgar score, serum pH, or arterial oxygen and carbon dioxide levels with subsequent neonatal hearing loss has, however, not been demonstrable.[23] Also noteworthy is the observation that neonates who suffer hypoxic, ischemic, or hemorrhagic insults frequently have multiple motor and/or cognitive deficits, whereas sensorineural hearing loss is more often an isolated finding.

Hyperbilirubinemia is one potential neonatal insult that has been associated with sensorineural hearing impairment in the absence of additional neurologic disabilities.[24] Bilirubin encephalopathy in full-term infants is typically associated with total serum bilirubin concentrations > 20 mg/dL; such infants may demonstrate a moderate to severe bilateral hearing impairment that is typically most marked in the middle- to high-frequency range. This vulnerability of the neural auditory pathways, particularly the cochlear nucleus, to bilirubin toxicity has been well documented in experimental-animal models.[25] Lower serum levels of bilirubin may also affect hearing thresholds, as indicated by recent BAER studies showing reversible prolongation of central auditory conduction latencies in neurologically intact infants with modest elevations of bilirubin concentration at levels of 10 to 16 mg/dL.[26] Bergman et al,[10] using multivariate analysis, demonstrated high total bilirubin concentration to be the principal single factor showing a positive correlation with sensorineural hearing loss in hearing-impaired low-birth-weight NICU survivors. This same study documented a negative association between exchange transfusions and hearing loss, suggesting that early exchange transfusions may prevent sensorineural hearing impairment in some premature neonates by decreasing potentially ototoxic serum bilirubin levels. Although an isolated role for hyperbilirubinemia has not been clearly elucidated, it does appear that the ototoxic level of bilirubin elevation in premature infants remains undefined and that the > 20 mg/dL level used for otherwise-healthy term infants is probably not applicable in this population.

Meningitis is stated to be the leading cause of acquired deafness in childhood.[3] The principal bacterial agents of meningitis in the older pediatric population—*Haemophilus influenzae*, *Neisseria meningitidis*, and *Streptococcus pneumoniae*—are infrequent in newborns. Group B streptococci and *Escherichia coli* strains account for about 70% of neonatal meningitis cases; *Listeria monocytogenes* is responsible for an additional 5% of cases.[27] Incidence rates are approximately 2 to 4 cases per 10,000 live births and may be as high as 1 case per 1,000 live births in some nurseries. The mortality is high, approximating 20% to 50%. Both short-term and long-term sequelae of neonatal meningitis are frequent, affecting 40% to 50% of surviving infants. The exact incidence of moderate to severe hearing impairment following neonatal meningitis has not been determined as specifically as in later-childhood cases. Five to thirty-five percent of children with childhood meningitis are estimated to suffer secondary sensorineural hearing loss; this incidence depends, in part, on the etiologic organism.[28]

Various other perinatal factors—maximum days of respiratory therapy, hypothermia, hyponatremia, hyperosmolarity, hypoglycemia, hypocalcemia, and diuretic therapy and other medical and surgical interventions—have been investigated as possible etiologies of neonatal sensorineural hearing loss. A concept has progressively developed of assigning perinatal risk for sensorineural hearing loss by means of a global assessment of health and therapy rather than attempting to correlate single, potentially ototoxic factors with eventual hearing status.[11,29,30] Although moderate to severe hearing impairment in NICU survivors is associated with some of these adverse perinatal events, no factor is absolute. The increased susceptibility of NICU graduates for sensorineural hearing loss is probably dependent on an interaction of both child-specific and NICU-specific factors. Whether the child-specific factors responsible for the neonate's admission to the NICU or care-specific factors of the NICU environment are the more important of these two remains undetermined. It simply can be said that graduation from an intensive-care nursery identifies an infant as being at high risk for sensorineural hearing impairment.

In 1982, the Joint Committee on Infant Hearing of the American Academy of Pediatrics developed criteria to identify newborns at risk for hearing loss[31]; a 1990 position statement expands these risk criteria[32] [see **Appendix A**]. The success of screening programs incorporating "high-risk" questionnaires is evident from the fact that the prevalence of moderate to profound sensorineural hearing loss in the original designated group of newborns is estimated to be 2.5% to 5.0%, figures 25- to 50-fold greater than for the pediatric population at large.

As a final note, many neonatal-hearing screening programs have identified a false-positive group of infants who fail their initial BAER screen but pass on subsequent testing.[8,9,33,34] Concomitant middle ear effusion with secondary conductive hearing loss that clears between testing sessions has been offered as one possible explanation for this observation.[35] Inspissated middle ear amniotic fluid may have a similar, temporary, conductive hearing effect.[36] Transient neurologic abnormalities in the neonatal population such as those secondary to hyperbilirubinemia[10,25] could also account for initial false-positive results on screenings for sensorineural hearing loss.

References
1. Schein JD, Delk MT Jr: *The Deaf Population of the United States*. Silver Spring, Md: National Association of the Deaf, 1974, p 16.
2. Fraser GR: The genetics of deafness, in Evans JNG (ed): *Pediatric Otolaryngology*. London: Butterworth & Co, 1987, pp 26-34.
3. Robillard TAJ, Gersdorff MCH: Prevention of pre- and perinatal acquired hearing defects: I. Study of causes. *J Aud Res* 1986;26:207.
4. Strauss M: A clinical pathologic study of hearing loss in congenital cytomegalovirus infection. *Laryngoscope* 1985;95:951.
5. Williamson WD, Percy AK, Yow MD, et al: Asymptomatic congenital cytomegalovirus infection: Audiologic, neuroradiologic, and neurodevelopmental abnormalities during the first year. *Am J Dis Child* 1990;140:1365.
6. Stennert E, Schulte FJ, Vollrath M, et al: The etiology of neurosensory hearing defects in preterm infants. *Arch Otorhinolaryngol* 1978;221:171.
7. Schulman-Galambos C, Galambos R: Brain stem evoked response audiometry in newborn hearing screening. *Arch Otolaryngol* 1979;105:86.
8. Sanders R, Durieux-Smith A, Hyde M, et al: Incidence of hearing loss in high risk and intensive care nursery infants. *J Otolaryngol* 1985;suppl 14:28.
9. Kramer SJ, Vertes DR, Condon M: Auditory brainstem responses and clinical follow-up of high-risk infants. *Pediatrics* 1989;83:385.
10. Bergman I, Hirsch RP, Fria TJ, et al: Cause of hearing loss in the high risk premature infant. *J Pediatr* 1985;106:95.
11. Duara S, Suter CM, Bessard KK, Gutberlet RL: Neonatal screening with auditory brainstem responses: Results of follow-up audiometry and risk factor evaluation. *J Pediatr* 1986;108:276.
12. Hendricks-Munoz KD, Walton JP: Hearing loss in infants with persistent fetal circulation. *Pediatrics* 1989;83:807.
13. Falk SA, Farmer JC Jr: Incubator noise and possible deafness. *Arch Otolaryngol* 1973;97:385.

14. Dayal VS, Kokshanian A, Mitchell DP: Combined effects of noise and kanamycin. *Ann Otol Rhinol Laryngol* 1971;80:897.
15. Jauhiainen T, Kohonen A, Jauhiainen M: Combined effect of noise and neomycin on the cochlea. *Acta Otolaryngol* 1972;73:387.
16. American Academy of Pediatrics Committee on Environmental Hazards: Noise pollution: Neonatal aspects. *Pediatrics* 1974;54:476.
17. Elfving J, Pettay O, Raivio M: A follow-up study on the cochlear, vestibular and renal function in children treated with gentamycin in the newborn period. *Chemotherapy* 1973;18:141.
18. Finitzo-Hieber T, McCracken GH Jr, Roeser RJ, et al: Ototoxicity in neonates treated with gentamycin and kanamycin: Results of a four-year controlled follow-up study. *Pediatrics* 1979;63:443.
19. Adelman C, Linder N, Levi H: Auditory nerve and brainstem evoked response thresholds in infants treated with gentamicin as neonates. *Ann Otol Rhinol Laryngol* 1989;98:283.
20. Sinha SK, D'Souza SW, Rivlin E, Chiswick ML: Ischaemic brain lesions diagnosed at birth in preterm infants: Clinical events and developmental outcome. *Arch Dis Child* 1990;65:1017.
21. Slack RW, Wright A, Michaels L, Frohlich SA: Inner ear cell loss and intracochlear clot in the preterm infant. *Clin Otolaryngol* 1986;11:443.
22. Vernon M: Clinical phenomenon of cerebral palsy and deafness. *Except Child* 1970;36:743.
23. Karjalainen S, Karja J, Suonio S, Yliskowski M: Intrauterine hypoxia as a cause of hearing impairment in children. *Int J Pediatr Otorhinolaryngol* 1982;4:233.
24. Keaster J, Hyman CB, Harris I: Hearing problems subsequent to neonatal hemolytic disease or hyperbilirubinemia. *Am J Dis Child* 1969;117:406.
25. Shapiro SM, Hecox KE: Brain stem auditory evoked potentials in jaundiced Gunn rats. *Ann Otol Rhinol Laryngol* 1989;98:308.
26. Perlman M, Fainmesser P, Sohmer H, et al: Auditory nerve-brainstem evoked responses in hyperbilirubinemic neonates. *Pediatrics* 1983;72:658.
27. McIntosh K: Bacterial infections of the newborn, in Avery ME, Taeusch HW Jr (eds): *Diseases of the Newborn*. Philadelphia: WB Saunders Co, 1984, pp 735-738.
28. Nadol JB: Hearing loss as a sequela of meningitis. *Laryngoscope* 1978;88:739.
29. Pettigrew AG, Edwards DA, Henderson-Smart DJ: Perinatal risk factors in infants with moderate-to-profound hearing deficits. *Med J Aust* 1988;148:174.
30. Salamy A, Eldredge L, Tooley WH: Neonatal status and hearing loss in high risk infants. *J Pediatr* 1989;114:847.
31. American Academy of Pediatrics Committee on Infant Hearing: Position statement. *Pediatrics* 1982;70:496.
32. Joint Committee on Infant Hearing 1990 position statement. *Head Neck Surg* 1991;10:15.
33. Shannon DA, Felix JK, Krumholz A, et al: Hearing screening of high-risk newborns with brainstem auditory evoked potentials: A follow-up study. *Pediatrics* 1984;73:22.
34. Durieux-Smith A, Picton TW, Edwards CG, et al: Brainstem electric response audiometry in infants of a neonatal intensive care unit. *Audiology* 1987;26:284.
35. Balkany TJ, Berman SA, Simmons MA, Jafek BW: Middle ear effusions in neonates. *Laryngoscope* 1978;88:398.
36. Northop C, Piza J, Eavey RD: Histological observations of amniotic fluid cellular content in the ear of neonates and infants. *Int J Pediatr Otorhinolaryngol* 1986;11:113.

Genetic Deafness and Hearing Impairment in Childhood

Kenneth M. Grundfast, MD

Points To Recall:
- Genetic hearing loss is a common reason for deafness.
- Clues for the etiology of the loss can occasionally be gleaned from the physical examination.
- Deafness is not always considered a disorder by some members of the deaf community.

Considerations for Referral:
- If a child has other family members with a hearing loss believed to be genetic
- If a child has findings on physical examination consistent with a genetic hearing loss

In recent years, several developments have brought about a new focus of attention and significance for inherited types of deafness within the spectrum of childhood hearing disorders. Inherited syndromes that include deafness have been newly discovered and reported, the genes causing some types of inherited deafness have already been located, and there is a great likelihood that experiments with cloned genes for inherited deafness will lead to a greater understanding of the genetic control of inner ear development and homeostasis.

Determining the incidence of genetic hearing loss is problematic, however, for several reasons. First, terms such as *deafness* and *hearing impairment* are not always clearly defined, and the incidence of the disorder varies in relationship to the definition of the disorder. The term *hearing impairment* may be used to describe disorders varying in severity from the mild conductive hearing loss associated with middle ear effusion in one ear to the bilateral profound sensorineural hearing loss, generally referred to as "complete deafness," that would be present in a child born with absence of both cochleae. In this paper, the terms *hearing impairment* and *deafness* are used interchangeably, with no connotation about severity implied with either term.

Second, in attempting to determine the incidence of genetic deafness, a distinction needs to be made between congenital and inherited disorders. *Congenital* means that a disorder is present at birth. *Inherited* means that the etiology of a disorder involves abnormal genes that code, via base-pair sequences, messages that result in abnormal development of cellular structures or degeneration of normally formed inner ear elements. Since there are many types of inherited deafness that characteristically do not begin to affect individuals until the 2nd or 3rd decade of life, we can see that inherited deafness does not have to be congenital. Conversely, the many infants who were born with deafness as a result of maternal rubella infection have congenital deafness that is not inherited.

Third, the likelihood that a case of childhood deafness will be classified as "inherited" depends, to a great extent, on the diligence with which a complete family history is ascertained. Often, there may be family members of an affected individual who have mild hearing impairment that is not known to other family members. Or known hearing impairments may have been attributed to such factors as infection, fever, trauma, or noise when the real underlying etiology of the hearing loss is genetic. Table 1 provides a summary of the parameters that can be used in describing genetic deafness of all types.

Table 1. Parameters in Description and Assessment of Genetic Deafness.

Terms used:	Hearing loss, hearing impairment, deafness
Time of onset:	Congenital, infancy, early childhood, adult life
Type:	Conductive, sensorineural, mixed
Severity:	Mild, moderate, severe, profound
Frequencies involved:	Low, middle, high
Stability:	Stable, fluctuating, progressive
Modes of inheritance:	Autosomal dominant, autosomal recessive, X-linked
Associated findings:	None (nonsyndromic), several (syndromic)

In a recent report, Cremers et al[1] analyzed results of eight previous studies on the etiology of childhood deafness in western Europe and Great Britain. In about half the cases, the hearing impairment was an isolated inherited disorder or part of an inherited syndrome. Approximately 1 person per 1,000 in a population of economically advantaged individuals will have hearing impairment severe enough to interfere with normal speech development.[2] In about 35% to 50% of congenitally deaf infants, the deafness is attributed to genetic factors, and about one third of these cases have associated anomalies that are recognizable as a syndrome.[3] About 80% of inherited deafness is transmitted in the autosomal recessive pattern and 20% is autosomal dominant. X-linked recessive deafness is rare. The autosomal dominant deafness varies more in severity and the degree to which associated anomalies are manifest than does the autosomal recessive type of deafness, which tends to have fewer associated anomalies and less variability in gene expression.

Making a Diagnosis

The five key factors in a physician's ability to make a diagnosis of genetic hearing loss are suspicion, most likely based on family history that an inherited disorder may exist; astute observations made during the physical examination; configuration of the audiogram; the physician's own fund of knowledge about the types of syndromic and nonsyndromic hearing disorders that can be inherited; and the ability to synthesize the information to formulate a diagnosis.

Suspicion

The most obvious situation in which inherited hearing loss would be suspected is when one or more members of a child's family are affected with hearing loss that has *not* been attributed to known etiologic factors such as infection, trauma, kernicterus, or any specific perinatal insult. For example, if a child is born into a family with a parent or sibling who has hearing impairment not known to have been "acquired," then there is a reasonable likelihood that the newborn child might also have hearing impairment. A different situation would be one in which family members all have normal hearing while possessing subtle findings recognizable as components of an inherited syndrome. For example, a child's father and grandfather might have ear pits and branchial cleft sinuses. In such a case, the child's physician should suspect hearing loss as part of the branchio-oto-renal syndrome.

Table 2 lists the questions that should be asked to elicit a history of inherited etiology when a child is diagnosed as having hearing impairment. In general, when sensorineural hearing loss is diagnosed in a child younger than 3 years of age and there is no obvious etiologic factor to explain the hearing impairment, then suspect that the etiology may be genetic.

Table 2. Questions To Elicit History Consistent With Genetic Deafness.

---

1. Are there any family members who were born with hearing impairment or who developed hearing impairment under the age of 30 years?
2. Are there family members who have pigmentary abnormalities such as premature gray hair or a white forelock of hair, two different-color eyes, widely spaced eyes, or hypopigmented areas of skin (Waardenburg syndrome)?
3. Are there family members who have hematuria, proteinuria, or kidney disorder?
4. Are there family members who have developed blindness?
5. Have there been syncopal episodes or cardiac arrhythmias?

Physical Examination

Abnormalities that might be associated with hearing loss are listed in Table 3. Identifying a constellation of findings as components of a syndrome can be viewed as a matter of pattern recognition. When a child has abnormalities that are obvious, then hearing loss would ordinarily be suspected if the findings are thought to fit a pattern identifiable as one of the syndromes that include hearing loss. However, more often than not, physical findings in a child or family member affected with inherited hearing loss may be subtle.

Table 3. Physical Examination of a Child With Newly Diagnosed Sensorineural Hearing Impairment.

1. *Face and head*: shape and symmetry, presence of skin tags
2. *Eyes*: shape, distance between eyes, slant of eyes, iris color, vision, eyegrounds
3. *Ears*: pinna shape, tortuosity/width/patency of external ear canal, pit/sinuses or skin tags in preauricular area
4. *Skin*: hyperpigmented areas, hypopigmented areas, café au lait spots
5. *Hair*: texture, color, white forelock
6. *Extremities*: carrying angle of arms, short or misshaped digits, extra digits, syndactyly
7. *Neck*: thyroid gland size, sinus tract orifices
8. *Other*: balance, gait

Audiologic Assessment

The audiogram can give clues to the diagnosis. The "cookie bite" shape audiogram (Figure), typically seen in individuals with inherited types of hearing impairment, has a characteristic configuration. Because the patient has better hearing in the low and high frequencies, the audiogram appears to have a bite taken out in the midfrequencies where the hearing is the worst.

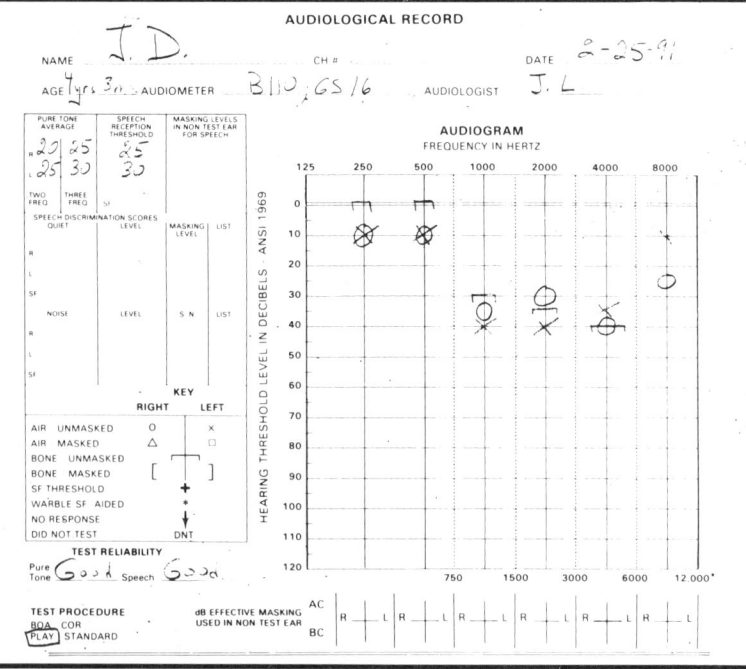

Figure. Example of a "cookie bite" audiogram.

Familiarity With Inherited Hearing Disorders

Two thirds of inherited hearing disorders are syndromic and one third are nonsyndromic. To make an accurate diagnosis, the physician needs to be familiar with and have access to a databank containing typical findings in the commonly occurring inherited hearing disorders. Although there are more than 200 inherited disorders that include hearing loss, many of the disorders are not common. Table 4 lists some of the commonly occurring inherited disorders that include hearing impairment.

Table 4. Commonly Occurring Types of Genetic Hearing Impairment.

With associated abnormalities (syndromic)
  Autosomal dominant
  - Treacher Collins syndrome (mandibulofacial dysostosis)
  - Goldenhar syndrome (facioauriculovertebral dysplasia)
  - Waardenburg syndrome
  - Branchio-oto-renal syndrome

  Autosomal recessive
  - Usher syndrome
  - Pendred syndrome
  - Jervell and Lange-Nielsen syndrome
  - Alport syndrome

Without associated anomalies (nonsyndromic)
  - Autosomal dominant delayed-onset progressive sensorineural hearing impairment
  - X-linked recessive mixed-stapes fixation with mixed hearing loss and perilymphatic gusher

Synthesis

Information obtained from the family history and pedigree analysis is combined with knowledge of the findings on physical examination and results of audiologic testing to determine if an individual is affected with inherited hearing impairment. Synthesis in diagnosis is really a matter of recognizing the significance of a particular constellation of findings. The recognizable pattern may consist of any combination of findings, including mode of inheritance, physical findings, characteristic appearance of an audiogram, timing of onset, and progression of hearing loss. For example, the findings of pigmentary abnormalities, widely spaced eyes, and variable types of sensorineural hearing impairment segregating among family members in an autosomal dominant mode of inheritance would be recognizable as Waardenburg syndrome. The association of congenital sensorineural hearing impairment with night blindness and abnormalities of the retina segregating in a family as an autosomal recessive trait would be recognizable as Usher syndrome.

Until recently, clinicians have attempted to arrive at a diagnosis of genetic deafness by taking a careful family history and being astute observers of subtle physical findings, then searching their memories in an attempt to match observed findings with a previously described disorder. Often, reference texts[2,4] have been helpful in matching findings with known disorders. Now, computer programs enable the user to enter data, including physical findings, audiologic test results, and inheritance patterns, to be matched with a diagnosis.[5]

Commonly Encountered Disorders

There are hundreds of inherited disorders that include hearing impairment; therefore, a primary-care physician cannot be expected to be familiar with all of them. On the other hand, a few inherited disorders occur relatively commonly. The primary physician could be familiar enough with characteristic findings (subtle or obvious) that a suspicion about the disorder will be raised during routine assessment of a child. Descriptions of some common inherited types of hearing impairment follow.

Facioauriculovertebral Dysplasia (Goldenhar Syndrome [Hemifacial Microsomia])

Typical findings include facial asymmetry due to underdevelopment of one mandibular ramus or condyle and a pinna abnormality that may be as slight as a protruding pinna or as severe as microtia. Preauricular skin tags and cervical vertebral dysplasia may be present. The hearing impairment is usually conductive.

Mandibulofacial Dysostosis (Treacher Collins Syndrome)

The hearing loss usually is more severe and more often bilateral than in Goldenhar syndrome. Typical findings include downward-slanting palpebral fissures, coloboma of the lower eyelids, malar hypoplasia, malformations of the external ear often associated with stenosis or atresia of the auditory canal, preauricular skin tags, dental malocclusion and teeth hypoplasia, and, sometimes, cleft palate or velopharyngeal incompetence. Recent evidence[6] suggests the gene for Treacher Collins syndrome is on chromosome 5.

Usher Syndrome

This condition is characterized by moderate to severe congenital deafness and retinitis pigmentosa, which develops in the 1st or 2nd decade of life. The inheritance pattern is autosomal recessive, and there is a possibility that carriers may be identified on the basis of abnormal vestibular function. Two types of the disorder have been described. The gene for Usher syndrome type II has been localized to chromosome 1q.[7]

Pendred Syndrome

This is another autosomal recessive disorder that includes congenital deafness and thyroid abnormalities. The thyroid gland may be enlarged and there may be some problems with thyroid hormone production; however, about 60% of affected individuals have normal thyroid function. The gene for Pendred syndrome has tentatively been located at chromosome 8q24.

Jervell and Lange-Nielsen Syndrome

This syndrome is characterized by congenital profound sensorineural deafness associated with syncopal episodes. Sudden death can occur in individuals whose cardiac conduction defect is evident as a prolonged Q-T interval and large upright, inverted, or biphasic T-waves.[8,9] Therefore, any deaf child who has syncopal episodes should have an ECG. This disorder may be seen in children attending schools for the deaf. Until recently, about half the children affected with this disorder died, probably of ventricular fibrillation, before age 15 years. However, now that children with the disorder can be treated with propranolol, the mortality rate has been reduced to less than 6%.

Stickler Syndrome

This condition is recognizable in children with marfanoid habitus who have severe myopia and prominent ankle, knee, and wrist joints and often have cleft palate, Pierre Robin sequence, and midface hypoplasia. These children may have progressive arthritis similar to juvenile rheumatoid arthritis. Retinal detachments and cataracts are seen frequently. The hearing loss can be conductive, sensorineural, or both. The inheritance pattern is autosomal dominant and there is considerable variability of expression.

Alport Syndrome

This disorder can be inherited as an autosomal dominant or X-linked trait. Patients have progressive symmetric sensorineural hearing loss with onset at about 20 years of age and nephritis with intermittent hematuria and proteinuria. The gene causing the X-linked type of the disorder has been mapped to Xq22-q25.[10]

Waardenburg Syndrome

This autosomal dominant pigmentary abnormality is associated with congenital hearing impairment. Characteristic findings include white hair forelock or premature graying of the hair, synophrys, and one iris with two different colors or two eyes of different colors. Patients with Waardenburg syndrome type I always have a wide space between the eyes; the gene for this type has been localized to chromosome 2q35-37.[11-13] The disorder may take many forms because of extremely high variation in expressivity of the gene.

Branchio-Oto-Renal Syndrome

This relatively common autosomal dominant type of genetic deafness is characterized by congenital hearing impairment, preauricular pits, branchial cysts or fistulae, and renal dysplasia that can be hypoplasia of a kidney or anomalies of the collecting system.[14]

X-Linked Recessive Mixed Deafness With Perilymphatic Gusher

This is one of the nonsyndromic inherited disorders that is not obvious on the basis of physical findings but would be evident if other family members had been affected. The hearing loss may be mild to severe, and an otologist who attempts to remove or mobilize a fixed stapes bone is likely to encounter a sudden rush of perilymphatic fluid from the vestibule of the inner ear.[15] The gene for this recessive form of deafness has not yet been localized, but clues to the location have been reported.[16]

Autosomal Dominant Delayed-Onset Progressive Sensorineural Deafness

This relatively common type of inherited hearing impairment is nonsyndromic, ie, not associated with obvious physical findings. The hearing loss is sensorineural, usually begins in the 2nd or 3rd decade, and often progresses to profound deafness involving both ears.

Diagnostic Studies

Although a diagnostic evaluation for sudden hearing loss in adults might be extensive and involve numerous metabolic studies, few diagnostic studies are helpful in the evaluation for genetic deafness. The studies that are recommended include urinalysis to check for proteinuria or hematuria, which might be a sign of Alport syndrome, and computed axial tomography to look for ossicular abnormalities of the middle ear or congenital abnormalities of the inner ear, such as the Mondini malformation. In addition, consultation with an ophthalmologist is advisable, especially if Usher syndrome is a diagnostic possibility. Consultation with a geneticist can help to determine whether the patient actually has a genetic type of hearing impairment. If an enlarged thyroid is palpated, thyroid-function tests should be obtained.

As the genes for inherited types of deafness are mapped, cloned, and sequenced, DNA tests will become available and many forms of syndromic and nonsyndromic genetic deafness will be diagnosed by testing the blood of individuals who are suspected of having a particular disorder.

Role of the Primary-Care Physician

Primary-care physicians play an important role in the identification and management of inherited hearing impairment in children. In cases involving a child newly diagnosed as having sensorineural hearing loss, the primary-care physician should consider genetic factors in the etiology of the hearing impairment. As mentioned, suspicion of inherited factors is a key to making the correct diagnosis. Therefore, when a parent or caregiver suspects that a child is not hearing normally, the child should be referred to an audiologist experienced in testing the hearing of young children. With auditory evoked-response testing or conditioned-response audiometry, an assessment will be made and hearing thresholds determined. A hearing aid can be placed if necessary.

Once a hearing loss has been documented, the child should be referred to an otolaryngologist who is experienced in dealing with hearing-impaired children. The otolaryngologist and the primary-care physician should confer and share information with a clinical geneticist for the purpose of determining etiology of the hearing loss. If the child has a severe or profound hearing loss, questions will arise regarding the appropriateness of oral-aural communication, sign language, or mainstream education. If the hearing loss is genetic, the parents may have questions about the risk that future children or siblings will be affected.

Primary-care physicians should be aware that the birth of a deaf child has a significant impact on family dynamics. Raising the child can be stressful for the parents, who will require considerable help with decision-making. A number of organizations can provide helpful information to parents [see **Appendix B**].

Ethical and Cultural Considerations

Finally, every clinician who cares for patients with inherited deafness needs to be sensitive to some of the issues that are important to members of the deaf community. First, among members of that community, deafness is not necessarily considered a disease, disorder, or handicap. In fact, some individuals, mostly those who use sign language as the primary method of communication, take pride in being deaf. They may come from families with other deaf members, may have attended schools for the deaf, and may socialize primarily with other deaf individuals. Although they acknowledge that being deaf can be troublesome in a world in which other individuals speak and hear, they enjoy being part of a deaf culture.

Therefore, a physician who makes a diagnosis of inherited deafness in a child must be cautious not to offend the parents or other affected family members by assuming that they will be disappointed to learn that the child is deaf. Deaf parents may *prefer* to have deaf rather than hearing children. This being the case, genetic counseling for the parents of a child diagnosed with inherited deafness must be approached with sensitivity.

References

1. Cremers CWRJ, Rijn PM, Hageman MJ: Prevention of serious hearing impairment or deafness in the young child. *Proc R Soc Med* 1989;82:483.
2. Fraser GR: *The Causes of Profound Deafness in Childhood*. Baltimore: Johns Hopkins University Press, 1976, p xi.
3. Black FO, Bergstrom L, Downs M, Hemenway W: *Congenital Deafness*. Boulder, Colo: Colorado Associated University Press, 1971, p 3.
4. Konigsmark BW, Gorlin RJ: *Genetic and Metabolic Deafness*. Philadelphia: WB Saunders Co, 1976, pp xv-xx.

5. Winter RM, Baraitser M: *London Dysmorphology Database.* New York: Oxford University Press, 1990.
6. Dixon MJ, Read AP, Donnal D, et al: The gene for Treacher Collins syndrome maps to the long arm of chromosome 5. *Am J Hum Genet* 1991;49:17.
7. Kimberling WJ, Weston MD, Moller C, et al: Localisation of Usher syndrome type II to chromosome 1q. *Genomics* 1990;7:245.
8. Schwartz PJ, Periti M, Malliani A: The long Q-T syndrome. *Am Heart J* 1975;89:378.
9. Keating M, Atkinson D, Dunn C, et al: Linkage of cardiac arrhythmia, the long QT syndrome, and the Harvey *ras*-1 gene. *Science* 1991;252:704.
10. Barker DE, Hostikka SL, Zhou J, et al: Identification of mutations in the COL 4A5 collagen gene in Alport syndrome. *Science* 1990;248:1224.
11. Foy C, Newton V, Wellesley D, et al: Assignment of the locus for Waardenburg syndrome type I to human chromosome 2q37 and possible homology to Splotch mouse. *Am J Hum Genet* 1990;46:1017.
12. Asher JH, Morrell R, Friedman TB: Waardenburg syndrome (WS): The analysis of a single family with WSI mutation showing linkage to RFLP markers on human chromosome 2q. *Am J Hum Genet* 1991;48:43.
13. Ishikiriyama S, Tonoki H, Shibuya Y, et al: Waardenburg syndrome type I in a child with de novo inversion (2)(q35q37.3). *Am J Med Genet* 1989;33:505.
14. Cremers CWRJ, Thijssen HO, Fischer AJ, Marres EH: Otological aspects of the earpit-deafness syndrome. *ORL* 1981;43:223.
15. Nance WE, Setleff RC, McLeod A, et al: X-linked mixed deafness with congenital fixation of the stapedial footplate and perilymphatic gusher. *Birth Defects* 1971;7(4):64.
16. Bento RF, Miniti A: X-linked mixed hearing loss: Four case studies. *Laryngoscope* 1985;95:462.

Deafness in Children Related to Meningitis

Philip R. Dodge, MD

Points To Recall:
- *Sensorineural hearing impairment is the most common permanent sequela of bacterial meningitis, occurring in about 10% of infected infants and children. The incidence is highest with* S pneumoniae *(31%).*
- *The impaired hearing usually occurs early in the course of disease. It may disappear during hospitalization for the acute illness, but if it persists for 2 to 3 weeks, it almost always remains permanent.*
- *Usually the infection extends into the inner ear from the subarachnoid space even though an associated otitis media is present.*

Considerations for Referral:
- *Every patient with meningitis requires otologic evaluation and audiometric tests.*
- *In young infants, electric response audiometry is desirable. Hearing in older infants may be assessed by conventional methods.*
- *Language development demands early referral to an appropriate therapeutic team.*

Bacterial meningitis is a leading cause, if not the most common cause, of acquired deafness in infancy and childhood. The incidence of hearing impairment associated with meningitis varies in both retrospective and prospective studies from about 5% to more than 30%. In our own prospective study of acute bacterial meningitis in infants and children older than 1 month of age,[1] the incidence of hearing loss was reported as 10.3%, but on long-term follow-up two additional patients with mild unilateral hearing loss were found, yielding a corrected incidence of 11.4%.

In this study, we accepted all patients admitted to St Louis Children's Hospital with acute bacterial meningitis between January 1973 and July 1977. One hundred ninety-one children were entered into the study with an acute mortality rate of 2% (one child died 1 year later). Because of congenital deafness, two infants were excluded from our study. One hundred eighty-five patients were eligible for follow-up, but only 159 patients were evaluated by electric response audiometry during or following hospitalization.

Of considerable interest was the difference in the incidence of hearing impairment, depending on the organism responsible for the meningitis. Thirty patients were infected by the *Streptococcus pneumoniae* organism, yet 31% of these children had impaired hearing, either unilateral or bilateral. In contrast, 10.5% of 19 patients with *Neisseria meningitidis* infection and 6% of 118 patients with *Haemophilus influenzae* infection had sensorineural hearing loss as a consequence of their meningitis.

The audiologic assessment was carried out under the direction of Dr Hallowell Davis, who during the early phase of the study was assisting in the development of the apparatus for measuring the evoked potential responses, first at the cerebral level and subsequently from the brainstem level. The audiometric examinations became more sophisticated and reliable over the course of the study, and eventually it was possible to measure pure tone thresholds at 500, 1000, 2000, and 4000 Hz.

Mild hearing impairment associated with middle ear disease was encountered in about 16% of these 159 patients who had audiometric testing. Ten patients had a sensorineural hearing loss that was bilateral, whereas in nine children the hearing impairment was limited to one ear. Those with unilateral hearing loss were obviously less handicapped. Hearing aids were used by most of the patients with bilateral hearing loss.

In our study, almost all children had hearing loss as an isolated neurologic deficit. Hearing impairment of sensorineural origin occurred in only five patients in association with either mental retardation, epilepsy, persistent quadriparesis, or hemiparesis. An initial cerebral spinal fluid glucose concentration of < 20 mg/dL was also correlated with sensorineural hearing impairment, but there was no correlation of hearing impairment with the initial concentration of protein, polyribose-phosphate capsular antigen, or number of leukocytes in the cerebral spinal fluid. Furthermore, there was no correlation between sensorineural hearing loss and sex, age, race, specific antibiotic treatment, presence of subdural effusions, acute seizures, or persistent ataxia. Unexpectedly, there was no correlation between sensorineural hearing loss and the number of days the patient had been ill before admission, defined as days with fever, vomiting, decreased activity, or lethargy. In most instances, it was the impression that these signs probably reflected an associated or antecedent viral infection. Needless to say, it was impossible to state with certainty what specifically caused these antecedent signs or when the meningitis began. Only when there are meningeal signs or unequivocal evidence of central nervous system dysfunction can one predict with some confidence what the result of lumbar puncture will be.

Investigators here and abroad have addressed the question of when in the course of bacterial meningitis damage to the auditory system is sustained. The study of Vienny and colleagues[2] from western Switzerland is particularly informative. They were able to record brain-stem auditory evoked potentials in 51 children from the earliest phase of the disease, within about 48 hours of establishing a diagnosis of meningitis. In 35 cases (68.6%), hearing was normal. In 11 cases (21.6%), the evoked potential audiogram was abnormal at 48 hours, but by the time of discharge from the hospital, approximately 2 weeks later, all in this group had recovered normal hearing. However, in five cases (9.8%), the hearing impairment persisted and was present at discharge from the hospital. This is in agreement with our overall incidence of hearing impairment of 11.4%. In no instance did any of these Swiss children with impaired hearing at discharge subsequently recover hearing. The authors concluded that, in this group with persistent auditory impairment, damage had occurred very early and was irreversible from the onset. It is of some interest that all the children with a permanent hearing deficit in the Vienny study had suffered from *H influenzae* meningitis; two were younger than 2 years of age, but the other three patients ranged in age from 4 to 15 years.

Kaplan and colleagues[3] had similar experiences. They were able to evaluate 37 children with bacterial meningitis within 48 hours of admission. Four of their patients had impaired hearing detected at the time of admission. Two of these patients had *H influenzae* and two had *S pneumoniae* as the causative organisms. Two of the children had severe to profound hearing loss that persisted, whereas improvement occurred in the other two children. None of the patients developed disordered hearing later in the course of disease or subsequently during follow-up. Similar findings were reported from Chicago by Özdamar et al.[4] They found that four of seven patients (57%) with pneumococcal meningitis had sensorineural hearing loss, although one patient had normal hearing on follow-up months later.

In a study of 60 infants and children with bacterial meningitis, Muñoz et al[5] carried out a prospective study in Mexico City of 34 children with *H influenzae* meningitis treated with chloramphenicol and of 36 children with meningitis caused by other microorganisms and treated with ampicillin. The authors concluded that there was no difference between patients treated before or after 48 hours of illness. Some 41% of patients with *H influenzae* meningitis and 22% of those with meningitis caused by other organisms had some impairment of hearing in one or both ears on initial examination. When tested approximately 6 months later, all but 2 of the 18 patients with early hearing impairment had recovered normal hearing, although it is not clear from the report precisely when this occurred. If one assumes that it occurred during hospitalization, a permanent rate of hearing loss of 11% would be in keeping with the recent results of other investigators.

In relation to the onset of deafness in acute bacterial meningitis, the report of Abad et al[6] is of considerable interest. They reported the case of a 20-year-old man who had neck pain following minor trauma. Examination was unremarkable except for an inflamed pharynx, and cervical spine films were normal. He was treated with an injection of penicillin and oral penicillin V for a presumed throat infection. Two days later he was admitted to the hospital because of increasing hearing loss, which was determined to be bilateral and of the sensorineural type. He was afebrile and had no signs of meningeal irritation but had first-degree nystagmus in all directions of gaze. It was only on the 2nd day that the signs of meningitis appeared, confirmed by examination of his cerebral spinal fluid. The organism was *N meningitidis*. The hearing loss persisted, although 3 months later hearing in the right ear had improved somewhat.

Where in the auditory system the pathology resides that produces hearing impairment in meningitis is uncertain. Most of the otopathologic studies of patients dying during the acute illness suggest that the inner ear is the most likely site. However, there also is clear evidence that inflammatory cells may surround the 7th and 8th cranial nerves. In children, Eavey et al[7] studied the temporal bones in eight patients who died with acute bacterial meningitis. In each instance, there was significant disease of the inner ear and associated evidence of inflammation of the nerves in the perineural space. It could well be that the latter is responsible for some of the transient hearing impairment but that the inner ear disease is responsible for the permanent deafness. A curious fact is that impaired facial nerve function is uncommon in acute bacterial meningitis, rendering this conclusion suspect. From the work of Eavey et al it is quite clear that even though there is associated otitis media in infants and children, the infection does not spread directly in a contiguous fashion to the inner ear. Rather, the infection appears to gain entrance to the labyrinth by way of the subarachnoid space early in the course of the meningitic process. Igarashi et al,[8] in a study of the mastoid bone in five people with pneumococcal meningitis, including two infants, found essentially the same pathology. In one of their patients, however, it appeared that the infection had spread directly to the stria vascularis from the bloodstream. This was associated with hemorrhage, suggesting a vasculitis with infarction of vessels supplying the stria vascularis and associated structures.

The lack of availability of otopathology remote from the acute bacterial infection has compounded the uncertainties as to the primary site of pathology. Recent experiences with cochlear implants, however, have afforded considerable insight into the problem. In individuals with profound hearing loss, surgeons have found evidence of fibrosis, calcification, and even bone formation in the inner ear. The ossification can be extensive, as reported by Eisenberg et al.[9] Ossification was greatest in those who had had *S pneumoniae* meningitis. It is possible, by drilling through this bony tissue, to insert the stimulating electrodes into the scala tympani in some, but not all, cases. The character of the inner ear findings strongly supports the conclusion that a pyogenic infection, rather than simply a toxin, is responsible for this pathology. But this does not exclude the possibility that toxins may be the cause of a transient or mildly persistent hearing impairment. On the other hand, it could well be that some of the transient sensorineural hearing impairment might relate to toxic involvement more central in the auditory system.

Because the hearing loss occurs very early in the course of meningitis, it has been hypothesized that the killing of the bacteria by the body's defense mechanisms, possibly augmented by antimicrobial agents, results in a release of cytokines that are in some way involved in injuring neural tissue. Corticosteroids are known to prevent or at least impede this process, leading McCracken and his colleagues[10-12] to treat patients with dexamethasone at the time of or before infusion of antibiotics. The potential importance of this treatment can hardly be overstressed. Given the development of sensorineural dysfunction early in the course of meningitis, prophylaxis would appear to be the ideal approach. However, before recommending the universal use of dexamethasone, replication of McCracken's finding by others would seem prudent.[13,14]

Currently, a multicenter study is in progress that may or may not confirm these earlier results. Equally exciting, if not more so, is the development of effective vaccines to prevent invasive disease due to *H influenzae*. It appears that the currently available conjugate vaccines are effective during the early months of life when the infant is at greatest risk for meningitis and deafness.

Finally, the role of postnatal aseptic meningitis due to viral infections deserves brief comment. In his review of 304 cases of presumed viral meningitis, Nadol[15] failed to find a single example of hearing impairment. His findings are in accord with those of other large series, although certainly isolated examples of virus-associated deafness are recorded. The mumps and measles viruses have been especially incriminated. In contrast to the seeming paucity of cases of deafness complicating viral meningitis during childhood and beyond, intrauterine viral infections are well known to devastate the auditory system. Rubella and cytomegaloviruses (CMVs) are especially prone to do this. Fortunately, immunization programs have all but eliminated the congenital rubella syndrome, including deafness. Recently, acquired hearing impairment from CMV has been encountered in persons with human immunodeficiency virus infection.

References

1. Dodge PR, Davis H, Feigin RD, et al: Prospective evaluation of hearing impairment as a sequela of acute bacterial meningitis. *N Engl J Med* 1984;311:869.
2. Vienny H, Despland PA, Lutschg J, et al: Early diagnosis and evolution of deafness in childhood bacterial meningitis: A study using brainstem auditory evoked potentials. *Pediatrics* 1984;73:579.
3. Kaplan SL, Catlin FI, Weaver T, Feigin RD: Onset of hearing loss in children with bacterial meningitis. *Pediatrics* 1984;73:575.
4. Özdamar O, Kraus N, Stein L: Auditory brainstem responses in infants recovering from bacterial meningitis: Audiologic evaluation. *Arch Otolaryngol* 1983;109:13.
5. Muñoz O, Benitez-Diaz L, Martinez MC, Guiscafre H: Hearing loss after *Hemophilus influenzae* meningitis: Follow-up study with auditory brainstem potentials. *Ann Otol Rhinol Laryngol* 1983;92:272.
6. Abad VC, Ng B, Somasunderam M: Hearing loss as an initial symptom of meningococcal meningitis. *Arch Neurol* 1983;40:451.
7. Eavey RD, Gao Y-Z, Schuknecht HF, González-Pineda M: Otologic features of bacterial meningitis of childhood. *J Pediatr* 1985;106:402.
8. Igarashi M, Saito R, Alford BR, et al: Temporal bone findings in pneumococcal meningitis. *Arch Otolaryngol* 1974;99:79.
9. Eisenberg LS, Luxford WM, Becker TS, House WF: Electrical stimulation of the auditory system in children deafened by meningitis. *Otolaryngol Head Neck Surg* 1984;92:700.
10. Lebel MH, Freij BJ, Syrogiannopoulos GA, et al: Dexamethasone therapy for bacterial meningitis: Results of two double-blind, placebo-controlled trials. *N Engl J Med* 1988;319:964.
11. Sáez-Llorens X, Ramilo O, Mustafa MM, et al: Molecular pathophysiology of bacterial meningitis: Current concepts and therapeutic implications. *J Pediatr* 1990;116:671.
12. Mustafa MM, Ramilo O, Sáez-Llorens X, et al: Cerebrospinal fluid prostaglandins, interleukin 1β, and tumor necrosis factor in bacterial meningitis: Clinical and laboratory correlations in placebo-treated and dexamethasone-treated patients. *Am J Dis Child* 1990;144:883.
13. Committee on Infectious Diseases, American Academy of Pediatrics: Dexamethasone therapy for bacterial meningitis in infants and children. *Pediatrics* 1990;86:130.
14. Schaad UB, Suter S, Gianella-Borradori A, et al: A comparison of ceftriaxone and cefuroxime for the treatment of bacterial meningitis in children. *N Engl J Med* 1990;322:141.
15. Nadol JB: Hearing loss as a sequela of meningitis. *Laryngoscope* 1978;88:739.

Discussion

Dr Cunningham: Dr Grundfast, do you obtain CT scans in all children in whom you newly diagnose sensorineural hearing loss, regardless of severity or pattern of loss?

If a child has a normal pediatric examination and appears to have isolated sensorineural hearing loss, do you obtain a genetic evaluation? What criteria do you use to help you in that regard?

Dr Grundfast: As a general rule, I don't use CT scanning in infants; it is just a matter of risk/benefit: some amount of radiation versus what I would do with the information in infancy.

I tend to use CT scans in children 5 years of age or older with no apparent etiology for the deafness. I look for inner ear abnormalities, such as Mondini deformity. I also look for a widened vestibular aqueduct, which has been reported in the last 5 years and which we are finding with increasing frequency in patients with no apparent etiology for sensorineural deafness—again, in children 5 years of age and older.

Dr Luxford: I think CT scans are needed earlier than 5 years of age. If you consider a profound hearing loss, the CT scan offers the possibility of defining a malformation, which provides information for prognosis. For example, if there is some kind of bone growth in the cochlea, the CT scan may offer information about use of a cochlear implant as early as age 2 years.

Dr Grundfast: In regard to genetic evaluation, the more time you spend training yourself to be an observer of physical findings that are known to be associated with genetic disorders (eg, of the face, pinna, eyes, extremities), and the more you train yourself to be a perceptive and astute historian in terms of family pedigree, the less you need to refer those patients to a geneticist initially, because the geneticist, to some degree, will be doing the same things you are.

I refer to a geneticist if I cannot fit the pattern together or if I suspect a pattern and need confirmation. Another reason to refer to a geneticist is that if you are fairly certain you have a pattern and are on your way to making a diagnosis of Treacher Collins syndrome or Goldenhar syndrome, then there are multisystem disorders. For example, in Goldenhar syndrome, you will look for vertebral and maybe renal abnormalities.

I believe that the best management for the patient involves three individuals at that point: the otolaryngologist, who will help with the ear and hearing disorders, the primary-care physician, who will help with the family and siblings and other aspects of management, and the geneticist, who is best able to determine which studies are necessary and how to handle the ongoing management.

Dr Ruben: The genetic work-up should include an evaluation of all the relatives who are available, especially older or younger siblings. If possible, the records of deceased members of the family should also be obtained. Many times, in cases of nonsyndromic hearing loss, an unsuspected family member will be identified with a hearing loss.

Dr Yaffe: Dr Cunningham, a question about newborn infants: How vigorously has the reduction of noise levels in incubators been pursued? The incubator is a device that is regulated by the Food and Drug Administration.

Dr Cunningham: Regulations do exist, and there also are manufacturers' standards.

Dr Ruben: The recommendations for noise reduction have been implemented.

Dr Yaffe: So we here don't have to do anything with respect to this type of noise.

Dr Brookhouser: There is more than just the background noise and the machinery in the nursery. There ought to be a general movement to try to quiet down the NICU. I am not necessarily saying the present noise level is potentially injurious, but I think making it quieter is important.

Another point we should stress to our primary-care colleagues is the importance of parental concern. This is an important high-risk indicator during the 1st year of well-baby care. One cannot afford to ignore a parent who thinks something is wrong with the child's hearing, and with the screening devices available today, one need not wait until a child outgrows the problem or it has been observed over a period of time.

Ototoxicity
Jo-Ann S. Harris, MD

Points To Recall:
- *To minimize the risk of ototoxicity, carefully evaluate the need to use any potentially ototoxic drug.*
- *Avoid the use of combination therapy with more than one potentially ototoxic drug.*
- *When using a potentially ototoxic drug, monitor serum concentrations of the drug and adjust the dosage accordingly.*

Considerations for Referral:
- *Periodic auditory and/or vestibular testing is recommended for children who receive ototoxic drugs and have preexisting sensorineural hearing loss, renal impairment, and elevated serum levels or who receive prolonged therapy, higher than ordinary doses, and more than one ototoxic drug, and children suspected to have cochlear or vestibular toxicity.*

Drug-induced ototoxicity is the result of damage to the cochlear or vestibular portions of the inner ear. Cochlear symptoms of ototoxicity include tinnitus and hearing loss, whereas vestibular symptoms consist of lightheadedness, giddiness, and vertigo. These symptoms can be transient or permanent, dose-related or idiosyncratic. Hearing loss secondary to drug ototoxicity is sensorineural and can be bilateral or unilateral.[1,2] Before World War II, reports of drug-induced ototoxicity involved mainly the salicylates and the antimalarial quinine. Drug-induced ototoxicity became more widely recognized after the discovery of the aminoglycoside streptomycin in 1944, which showed significant ototoxicity, mainly vestibular, in patients being treated for tuberculosis.[3] Since that time, the numerous aminoglycoside antibiotics now in widespread use have shown varying degrees of ototoxicity. Many other classes of drugs have also been implicated, including other nonaminoglycoside antibiotics, loop diuretics, antimalarials, salicylate-containing products, and anticancer chemotherapeutic agents.

This paper focuses on the drugs with ototoxic potential that are commonly used in infants and children and presents information on monitoring children who are taking these drugs to help minimize the risk of hearing loss.

The drugs with potential ototoxicity that are most commonly used in infants and children are listed in Table 1. The aminoglycoside antibiotics are the most frequently used and best-studied of these drugs. The other drugs of particular interest in children include vancomycin, erythromycin, furosemide, and cisplatin.

Table 1. Potentially Ototoxic Drugs Commonly Used in Infants and Children.

Aminoglycoside Antibiotics	Antimalarials
Kanamycin	Chloroquine phosphate
Gentamicin	Quinine sulfate
Tobramycin	Loop Diuretic
Amikacin	Furosemide
Netilmicin	Salicylate
Neomycin	Aspirin
Other Antibiotics	Other
Vancomycin	Cisplatin
Erythromycin	

Aminoglycosides

The aminoglycoside antibiotics are frequently prescribed for empiric therapy of sepsis and meningitis in newborn infants, suspected sepsis in oncology patients, respiratory infection in patients with cystic fibrosis, intra-abdominal sepsis, wound infections in burn patients, and infections due to gram-negative bacilli in the blood, cerebrospinal fluid, and urine.[4] Aminoglycosides are poorly absorbed orally, are not metabolized, and are excreted primarily by glomerular filtration. The exact mechanism of ototoxicity is unknown. These drugs can concentrate in the perilymph and accumulate there with repetitive dosing. Accumulation in the perilymph can depend on amount of the administered dose, dosing interval, duration of treatment, and rate of elimination from the plasma.[5] The ototoxicity appears to result from damage to the outer hair cells of the cochlea, with high-frequency hearing loss appearing first, and damage to type I hair cells in the central region of the vestibulum.[4,5]

The various aminoglycosides differ in the extent and type of ototoxicity, ie, cochlear versus vestibular. Experimental studies in animals have shown kanamycin and amikacin to be most toxic to the cochlea, followed by gentamicin and then tobramycin, with netilmicin the least toxic. Streptomycin is the most toxic to the vestibular apparatus, followed by gentamicin, tobramycin, and amikacin, with netilmicin the least toxic.[4,5]

Although there have been numerous publications, mainly about adult patients, comparing ototoxicity of aminoglycosides, the overall incidence remains unclear. Kahlmeter and Dahlager[6] reviewed the clinical studies published from 1975 to 1982 involving 6,494 patients. They found the average incidence of cochlear toxicity to be 13.9% with amikacin, 8.3% with gentamicin, 6.1% with tobramycin, and 2.4% with netilmicin. Vestibular toxicity was reviewed in only 1,976 patients and was found in 3.2% and 3.5% treated with gentamicin and tobramycin, respectively, and in 2.8% and 1.4% treated with amikacin and netilmicin, respectively.

The incidence of ototoxicity in infants and children remains controversial, and it appears that pediatric patients may be more resistant than adults to the ototoxic effects of these drugs. Several extensive reviews of the pediatric literature have failed to show significant rates of ototoxicity.[4,5,7] Very few well-controlled prospective studies have been conducted with pediatric patients. Most studies used conventional audiometric tests that required cooperation of the patient and therefore were done after 2 years of age; only within the last decade has brainstem evoked-response audiometry (BERA) been used to evaluate ototoxicity, ie, cochlear function, in infants.[4] Vestibular function was usually not evaluated, as doing so is extremely cumbersome in infants. More recent prospective, well-controlled, longitudinal studies by Finitzo-Hieber et al[8,9] evaluating both cochlear and vestibular functions have shown a low risk of aminoglycoside-associated ototoxicity in neonates with netilmicin, amikacin, gentamicin, or tobramycin. Many factors have been proposed to increase the risk of aminoglycoside ototoxicity, and Table 2 lists those that may be of particular importance in infants and children.

Ototoxicity has been reported with fetal exposure to aminoglycosides. There is placental transfer of the drug, and experimental data show susceptibility to toxicity during the gestational period of onset of auditory function.[2,5] The cochlea is formed by the 23rd week of gestation. There are several case reports of ototoxicity in infants whose mothers were treated with streptomycin during pregnancy, the risk being greater with maternal renal failure or use of another ototoxic drug.[2,5] Ototoxicity in the fetus has not been well studied in humans and there has been no documentation of whether the fetal ear is more susceptible to damage. Age-related risk of aminoglycoside toxicity is due primarily to immature renal function. During the neonatal period, the glomerular filtration rate is immature, with maturity of renal function associated with gestational age. Glomerular filtration increases during the 1st month of life, although the increase is slower in premature and low-birth-weight infants; this accounts for the higher risk of drug accumulation in these infants. Although the drug disposition favors accumulation and therefore higher

Table 2. Possible Factors Associated With Increased Risk of Aminoglycoside Ototoxicity in Infants and Children.

Age	Use of Other Otoxic Drugs
Fetus[2,5,7]	Vancomycin[11]
Premature infant[7]	Loop diuretics[1,12]
Newborn[7]	Route of Administration
Underlying Clinical Condition[7]	Topical (eardrops)[13-15]
Apnea	Intrathecal
Hypoxia	Intraventricular
Hyperbilirubinemia	Total Dose[5,7,8]
Electrolyte imbalance	Peak-and-Trough Serum Levels
Hypotension	Familial Predisposition[7]
Sepsis/Meningitis	
Renal impairment[7]	
Noise	
Maintenance in incubator[2,4,10]	

serum concentrations in the neonate, it is counterbalanced by the larger volumes of distributions of drug. Renal impairment in infants and children does increase the risk of drug accumulation at all ages.[7]

The combination of noise and aminoglycoside antibiotics, in particular kanamycin and neomycin, has been shown to act synergistically to cause ototoxicity in experimental animals.[2,4,10] This becomes a matter of special concern for infants being maintained in incubators. The additive effect of noise and aminoglycosides has not been demonstrated in premature infants who receive drugs in incubators.

Several animal studies have shown a striking potentiation of ototoxicity with the use of loop diuretics and aminoglycosides, and the effect appears to be additive.[12] Furosemide alone has been shown to have an incidence of ototoxicity as high as 6%.[1] The serum half-life of furosemide is prolonged in premature infants due to hepatic and renal insufficiency. Although there have been several reports of deafness from use of loop diuretics in patients with previous or concomitant aminoglycoside therapy, clinical studies in adults have failed to show an increased risk of aminoglycoside ototoxicity.[16]

Indomethacin has been found to decrease glomerular filtration, and increased serum concentrations of aminoglycosides have been observed when these drugs are coadministered, although clinical ototoxicity has not been documented.[4]

Intrathecal and intraventricular routes of administration of aminoglycosides have been implicated in an increased risk of ototoxicity. These routes are no longer used in the treatment of neonatal meningitis and therefore are now of theoretic interest only. The route of administration that has stimulated the most controversy is topical, as for eardrops. Eardrops containing aminoglycoside antibiotics are a common treatment of chronic suppurative otitis media in children who have either a perforation of the tympanic membrane or tympanostomy tubes. In animal studies, when solutions containing aminoglycoside antibiotics are instilled into the middle ear, they cause severe cochlear damage, loss of hair cells, and resultant abnormal cochlear function.[13,14] Other solutions that showed cochlear toxicity in these animal models include drug vehicles (eg, propylene glycol), antiseptics, and chloramphenicol. Although there have been reports of ototoxicity in humans following use of topical eardrops,[13,15] clinical studies in general have not corroborated these animal-study findings.

Several theories have been proposed as to why there seems to be little documented ototoxicity in humans in the face of widespread use of aminoglycoside eardrops. First, chronic suppurative otitis may cause a hearing loss; to distinguish this from hearing loss due to eardrops becomes problematic. Second, absorption of drug into the inner ear may be decreased due to either the oblique orientation of the human round window or poor penetration through chronically infected middle ear tissue or both.[13,17] Clinicians are concerned about the ototoxic potential of topical eardrops. Some are recommending that they be used with caution in patients with perforated tympanic membranes and suggest maintaining close medical supervision of patients who are treated with eardrops[17] and considering alternative treatments for chronic suppurative otitis media.[18]

High daily and total doses of aminoglycosides as well as elevated peak-and-trough serum concentrations have been shown to increase the risk of ototoxicity in adults.[5,7,19] Studies in children are limited, but large doses, prolonged treatments, and decreased drug clearance, such as in patients with renal insufficiency, have also been found to be risk factors for ototoxicity in children.[5,7]

Familial predisposition for ototoxicity has been reported[7] in two studies of families being treated with streptomycin for tuberculosis. This phenomenon has not been reported for other aminoglycosides.

Vancomycin and Erythromycin

Vancomycin

Although there have been reports of hearing loss associated with vancomycin, particularly when serum concentrations exceed 45 mg/L,[17] the ototoxicity of vancomycin has not been well established and is, in fact, questionable. There are no reports of ototoxicity of vancomycin in experimental animals. The original reports of ototoxicity were most likely a result of impurities in the early vancomycin preparations. The few more-recent reports of ototoxicity have only been in patients who also received an aminoglycoside antibiotic just before, during, or after the vancomycin. It has been shown in animals that vancomycin enhances the ototoxicity of aminoglycosides.[11] Premature infants may be at increased risk for any potential toxicity because of the longer serum half-life of vancomycin.

Erythromycin

Erythromycin ototoxicity was first noted in patients being treated for legionella pneumonia. The symptoms of tinnitus, vertigo, and hearing loss are reversible, occur at high doses (ie, > 2 g/day given intravenously), and generally are seen in elderly patients with hepatic or renal dysfunction.[11] Information on ototoxicity in children is lacking.

Cisplatin

Both vestibular toxicity and cochlear toxicity have been described with cisplatin, a commonly used anticancer chemotherapeutic agent. Rates of toxicity range as high as 20%, but the exact incidence is difficult to define. Bilateral hearing loss is the most common sign of ototoxicity, with high-frequency hearing loss appearing first.[1,17] Toxicity is related to total dose (ie, > 3 to 4 mg/kg or 100 mg/m^2), and children receiving high doses of cisplatin (> 540 mg/m^2) have a high incidence of hearing loss that appears to be potentiated by cranial irradiation.[1] Ototoxicity may be minimized by using slow infusion and divided doses.

Monitoring Children on Ototoxic Drugs

To minimize the risk of ototoxicity, it is important to evaluate the need for a potentially ototoxic drug and to determine whether a suitable alternative is available. It is also important to avoid the use of combination therapy with more than one potentially ototoxic drug. Any predisposing factors associated with increased risk of ototoxicity should be taken into account when establishing treatment and follow-up plans. When using a potentially ototoxic drug, it is important to monitor serum concentrations of the drug and adjust the dosage accordingly. This is especially true for the aminoglycosides and vancomycin, as serum drug-level testing is readily available at most clinical laboratories.

Table 3 lists some guidelines for desirable serum concentrations of aminoglycosides and vancomycin in children. It is important to obtain peak-and-trough serum concentrations of aminoglycoside antibiotics if there is any concern about altered drug disposition, as in premature and very-low-birth-weight infants and in children with renal impairment. In addition, measuring serum concentrations of aminoglycoside antibiotics is recommended when 1) therapy is longer than 3 days, 2) the patient is receiving more than one potentially ototoxic drug, 3) the patient requires higher than ordinary doses, eg, for cystic fibrosis, and 4) there is any clinical evidence of ototoxicity. Generally, the first set of peak-and-trough levels is obtained within the first 3 days of therapy and the levels are monitored once or twice a week thereafter, depending on the circumstances of the individual patient.

Recommendations for when to refer the child for auditory and/or vestibular testing[17] are listed in Table 4. In certain circumstances, it may be necessary to refer the child for baseline testing before initiation of therapy with a potentially ototoxic drug such as cisplatin.

Table 3. Guidelines for Desirable Serum Concentrations of Aminoglycosides and Vancomycin in Children.

Drug	Desirable Serum Concentration (μg/mL) Peak[a]	Trough[b]	Potentially Toxic Range (μg/mL)
Gentamicin	5-10	< 2	> 14
Tobramycin	5-10	< 2	> 14
Kanamycin	20-35	< 10	> 40
Amikacin	20-35	< 10	> 40
Vancomycin	15-30	< 10	> 40

[a]Peak levels drawn 1-2 hours after administration
[b]Trough levels drawn within 15-30 minutes before next dose

Table 4. Monitoring Children on Ototoxic Drugs.

Periodic Auditory and/or Vestibular Testing Is Recommended for Children With:
- Preexisting sensorineural hearing loss
- Renal impairment
- Elevated serum levels of an ototoxic drug
- Prolonged therapy on an ototoxic drug
- Higher than ordinary doses of an ototoxic drug
- Therapy with more than one ototoxic drug
- Evidence of cochlear and/or vestibular toxicity

References
1. Rybak LP, Matz GJ: Ototoxicity, in Rubin R, Alberto P (eds): *Otologic Medicine and Surgery*. New York: Churchill Livingstone, 1988, pp 1623-1635.
2. D'Alonzo BJ, Cantor AB: Ototoxicity: Etiology and issues. *J Fam Pract* 1983;16:489.
3. Hawkins JE: Introduction: Historical perspective, in Lerner SA, Matz GJ, Hawkins JE (eds): *Aminoglycoside Ototoxicity*. Boston: Little Brown & Co, 1981, pp xvii-xx.
4. McCracken GH: Aminoglycoside toxicity in infants and children. *Am J Med* 1986;80(suppl 6B):172.
5. Assael BM, Parini R, Rusconi F: Ototoxicity of aminoglycoside antibiotics in infants and children. *Pediatr Infect Dis* 1982;1:357.
6. Kahlmeter G, Dahlager JI: Aminoglycoside toxicity: A review of clinical studies published between 1975 and 1982. *J Antimicrob Chemother* 1984;13(suppl A):9.
7. Siegel JD, McCracken GH: Aminoglycoside ototoxicity in children, in Lerner SA, Matz GJ, Hawkins JE (eds): *Aminoglycoside Ototoxicity*. Boston: Little Brown & Co, 1981, pp 341-353.
8. Finitzo-Hieber T, McCracken GH, Roeser RI, et al: Ototoxicity in neonates treated with gentamicin and kanamycin: Results of a four-year controlled follow up study. *Pediatrics* 1979;63:443.

9. Finitzo-Hieber T, McCracken GH, Brown KC: Prospective controlled evaluation of auditory functions in neonates given netilmicin or amikacin. *J Pediatr* 1985;106:129.
10. Bhattacharyya TK, Dayal VS: Ototoxicity and noise-drug interaction. *J Otolaryngol* 1984;13:361.
11. Brummett RE, Fox KE: Vancomycin and erythromycin induced hearing loss in humans. *Antimicrob Agents Chemother* 1989;83:791.
12. Brummett RE: Effects of antibiotic-diuretic interactions in the guinea pig model of ototoxicity. *Rev Infect Dis* 1981;3(suppl):S216.
13. Morizono T: Ototopical agents: Ototoxicity in animal studies. *Ann Otol Rhinol Laryngol* 1988;97(suppl 131):28.
14. Brummett RE, Harris RF, Lindgren JA: Detection of ototoxicity from drugs applied topically to the middle ear space. *Laryngoscope* 1976;86:1177.
15. Podoshin L, Fradis M, Ben David J: Ototoxicity of ear drops in patients suffering from chronic otitis media. *J Laryngol Otol* 1989;103:46.
16. Moore RD, Smith CR, Lietman PS: Risk factors for the development of auditory toxicity in patients receiving aminoglycosides. *J Infect Dis* 1984;149:23.
17. Matz GJ: Clinical perspectives on ototoxic drugs. *Ann Otol Rhinol Laryngol* 1990;99:39.
18. Kenna MA, Bluestone CD, Reilly JS: Medical management of chronic suppurative otitis media without cholesteatoma in children. *Laryngoscope* 1986;96:146.
19. Siegenthaler WE, Bonetti A, Luthy R: Aminoglycoside antibiotics in infectious diseases: An overview. *Am J Med* 1986;80(suppl):2.

Loud Sound: Ear Damage, Hearing Loss, and Ear Protection

M. Charles Liberman, PhD

Points To Recall:
- *A typical audiogram pattern of noise-induced hearing loss demonstrates a loss initially in the 4-6 kHz range.*
- *Children can come into contact with environmental noise that can potentially damage hearing.*
- *Ear protectors can preserve hearing.*

Considerations for Referral:
- *Patient or parental concern about hearing loss*
- *Tinnitus that does not subside*
- *Patients at risk, eg, those who work with loud farm machinery, sport-rifle hunters, rock-band musicians*

Basic Noise Measurement

The sensation of hearing results from rapidly changing sound-pressure waves impinging on our ears. The operating range of the human ear is immense: The amplitude of a just-detectable sound is 10,000,000 times smaller than the amplitude that first causes a painful sensation. Because of this enormous range, sound levels are described on a logarithmic scale known as the decibel scale. Zero-dB sound-pressure level (SPL) is defined to be the threshold of human hearing, and corresponds to an absolute value of 0.0002 dynes/cm^2. As a rule of thumb, the perceived loudness of a sound doubles with each 10-dB increase in stimulus intensity.

One of the simplest of sounds is the pure tone, such as that produced by a tuning fork, which corresponds to a sinusoidal variation of sound pressure over time. The frequency of a tone is simply the number of pressure peaks (or troughs) per second. The human ear is responsive to tones from frequencies of 50 Hz (cycles per second) to about 20,000 Hz. "Middle C" corresponds to 256 Hz, while the highest note on the piano is about 4500 Hz, well below the high-frequency limit of normal hearing.

Most sounds in our environment are complex; that is, they are made up of many frequency components. Just as visible light can be described as the sum of many wavelengths across the spectrum between infrared and ultraviolet, any complex noise can be analyzed into its component frequencies and their relative amplitudes. Some noises, such as a teakettle whistle, are composed primarily of high-frequency sounds, while others, such as those from a poorly muffled car, are predominantly low frequency. We can measure the overall sound pressure of a complex sound, representing the summed pressure of all the component frequencies. However, both the frequency content and intensity level of a sound are important in determining its damage potential.

Noise-Induced Structural Damage to the Ear

Virtually all structures of the middle and inner ears can be damaged by sound if the intensity is made high enough. However, the middle ear is damaged only by sound pressures in excess of 160 dB, such as those produced by high-intensity impulse noises (eg, bomb blasts). The most common middle ear damage is eardrum rupture, which can be surgically repaired if it fails to heal spontaneously.

As illustrated in Fig 1, the more common noises in our environment are of significantly lower intensities than those achieved by dangerous impulsive stimuli. Ear damage from these less extreme noises is almost always confined to the inner ear, where it is the sensory cells themselves, called *hair cells*, that appear to be the most vulnerable. Overstimulation by loud sounds can cause swelling of the hair cells and even herniation of their apical surfaces. These apical "blisters" sometimes envelop the sensory hairs ("stereocilia") anchored there. Damage to the stereocilia remains even if the cellular swelling subsides. Alternatively, the apical blisters may burst, in which case the sensory cell dies. Following cell death, the nerve fibers contacting it usually degenerate within a few months.[1] Each human ear contains roughly 16,000 sensory cells and 30,000 nerve fibers at birth. Once a hair cell or nerve fiber is lost, it is not replaced, and any resulting hearing loss is therefore permanent.

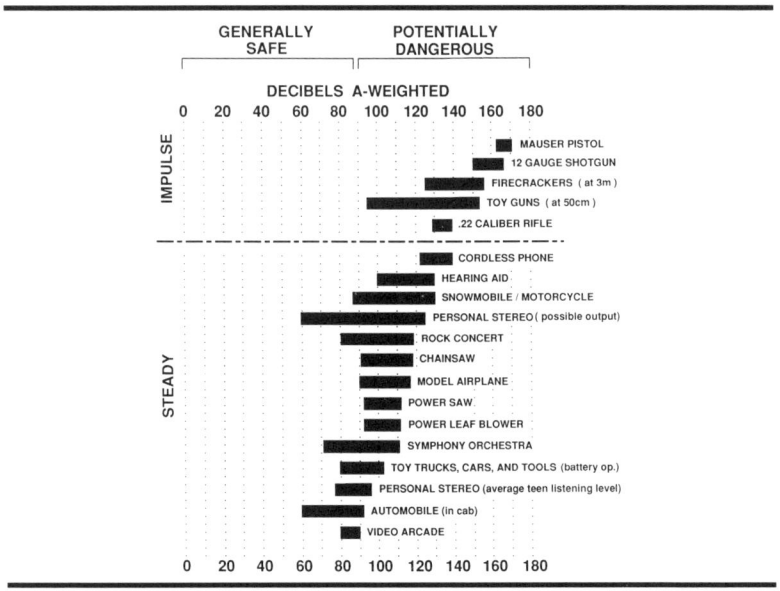

Fig 1. Intensity of example environmental sounds.

Noise-Induced Hearing Loss: Basic Features

Threshold shift is typically worst at midfrequencies. The classic audiometric pattern for noise-induced hearing loss (NIHL) is the so-called 4-kHz notch, ie, maximum deficit at frequencies near 4 to 6 kHz (4000-6000 Hz). As the severity of the loss worsens, the threshold shift spreads to the high frequencies (8-16 kHz) much more than to the low (0.25-2.0 kHz).[2] This audiometric pattern arises because of two complementary tendencies: 1) The damage potential of a sound increases with increasing frequency, yet 2) most high-intensity noise sources in our environment have maximum energy at low frequencies and steadily decreasing energy at higher frequencies. The tendency for these opposing trends to produce maximum damage at midfrequencies is reinforced by the natural resonance of the human ear canal at roughly 4 kHz, which tends to selectively amplify sounds in that frequency range.

Hearing deteriorates only as long as the exposure continues. NIHL can be measured immediately after the termination of the exposure and can occur following a single exposure incident if the sound pressure is high enough (> ~ 125 dB). Repeated audiometric testing after the exposure shows a period of improvement followed by a period of stabilization. Postexposure deterioration in hearing is almost never seen.

Hearing can improve for as long as a month postexposure. Recovery of hearing levels following overexposure occurs along an exponential time course; ie, improvement is by a constant percentage per hour, rather than by a constant decibel per hour. Thus the dB/hour improvement is constantly decreasing, and final hearing levels are approached asymptotically. This also means that the length of the postexposure recovery period is proportional to the severity of the hearing loss. Acute losses < 40 dB (measured within an hour of the exposure) often are recovered completely within a few days. Acute losses > 40 dB often result in some permanent deficit. However, only after several weeks of recovery do the hearing levels stabilize at final values.

NIHL is often associated with tinnitus. In addition to the sensation of hearing loss, overexposure to sound is also often associated with ringing in the ears, or tinnitus.[3] Tinnitus onset can be abrupt, as with hearing loss following an impulsive stimulus. In cases where the hearing loss is recovered, the tinnitus usually disappears. In cases of permanent NIHL, the tinnitus can also persist. It is often the tinnitus, rather than realization of a hearing loss, that causes a patient to seek medical attention.

There is tremendous intersubject variability in susceptibility to NIHL. Some people have "tough ears," whereas others have "tender ears." If a large group is exposed to an identical sound source, a wide range of hearing losses results: Some people are unaffected; others might have NIHLs of 40 to 60 dB. The extent to which susceptibility is correlated with age, sex, and race is controversial, and this intersubject variability complicates the process of defining safe versus dangerous levels of sound.

Defining Safe Versus Dangerous Exposures

Given the three independent variables of frequency, intensity, and time, an infinite variety of possible acoustic overexposures exist. It is, therefore, a daunting task to specify in some simple and reliable way which exposures are safe and which are dangerous. Nevertheless, certain summary statements can set the stage for a description of general "damage-risk criteria":

For uninterrupted exposures, noise-induced damage is roughly proportional to the total energy (duration × intensity) of the stimulus. Thus, if you double the intensity of the stimulus, you should cut the duration in half to expect the same damage.

For a given level of total exposure energy, an interrupted exposure is much less dangerous than an uninterrupted one. That is, rest periods are very important. Given a task that requires 8 hours at a noisy machine, attempting the job in one 8-hour day could result in NIHL, while performing it 2 hours/day for 4 days might be completely safe. Thus, noise exposures are not strictly cumulative over a lifetime in the same way that radiation exposure, for example, appears to be.

At a given intensity, high-frequency stimuli are more dangerous than low-frequency stimuli. In general, we have poorer hearing at frequencies below 1.0 kHz than above; that is, low-frequency sounds must be louder to be detected. Correspondingly, the "safe" intensity range extends to higher sound pressures for low-frequency sounds than for high. In keeping with this fundamental principle, noise measurements are more meaningfully expressed in the context of NIHL with the "A-weighted" dB scale, which filters the noise to deemphasize contributions from low-frequency components.

At a given overall intensity, narrow-band stimuli are more dangerous than broad-band stimuli. Concentrating a fixed amount of energy into a small frequency band (as is the case for a pure tone) results in higher maximum vibrations within the inner ear than if the energy is spread over many frequency bands. This concentration of energy is therefore capable of producing greater damage.

A sound need not be painful to cause permanent NIHL. The threshold of pain (roughly 140 dB) is well above the level at which sounds can be dangerous to the ear (approximately 90 dB with prolonged exposure). One cannot overemphasize the importance of this unfortunate fact.

With these basic principles in mind, the Occupational Safety and Health Administration (OSHA) has developed damage-risk criteria for exposure to steady-state noises, defined as those longer than 500 milliseconds in duration. Their purpose was to describe exposures that would leave most (although not all) people with normal hearing after at least 20 years of exposure, 5 days a week, 52 weeks a year. The resulting guidelines for "permissible" exposure doses over a range of A-weighted intensities are given in Fig 2. The maximum permissible level for impulse noises (those lasting < 500 ms) is 140 dB.

OSHA GUIDELINES FOR STEADY NOISES	
NOISE LEVEL dB (A)	ALLOWABLE DURATION (per day, 5 days/week)
90	8 hours
95	4 hours
100	2 hours
105	1 hour
110	30 minutes
115	15 minutes
120	7.5 minutes

Fig 2. OSHA guidelines for steady noises.

Examination of the A-weighted sound-pressure ratings in Fig 1 shows that a wide range of commonly pursued noisy activities put the hearing organ at risk. It is instructive to consider from which noises the hearing losses have been clearly documented.

Among the best-documented and most clear-cut causes of NIHL is exposure to explosive impulses such as gunfire or firecrackers. A number of studies of adult hunters show clearly that NIHLs > 40 dB can be seen following many years of "leisure" exposure to gunfire.[4] One study of 1,000 schoolchildren in India, with hearing tests performed before and after a national holiday in which firecracker use is rampant, showed that 5% suffered permanent NIHL.[5] Thus, for high-intensity impulsive exposures, the risks of hearing damage are very clear.

As for steady-state noise exposures in children, the risk factor that receives the most attention is exposure to loud music, either at rock concerts or through headphones of personal stereo systems. Although the peak sound pressures at a rock concert may reach 115 dB(A), the time-weighted average over a 1-hour "set" is closer to 100 dB(A),[6] at which level OSHA guidelines would allow exposure for 2 hours per day, 5 days a week. Thus, although temporary threshold shifts probably occur in a sizable fraction of the audience, such NIHL would typically recover within hours postexposure. Hearing levels in frequent versus infrequent attendees at rock concerts show no significant differences. Thus, although permanent NIHL may well be a problem for some music performers, there is no solid basis for alarm about audience safety.

The literature on personal stereo use shows that, although such devices are capable of producing very dangerous SPLs, most users (even teenagers listening to their rock favorites) choose levels below 100 dB(A). Nevertheless, a sizable fraction of young users listen for long-enough periods that their exposures significantly exceed OSHA guidelines.[7] Although definitive demonstration of significant NIHL from this activity has yet to be shown, such exposures may take years to exact their toll on the hearing organ, and the potential danger of this habit cannot be ignored. This is especially true given the spread of personal stereo use to younger and younger children.

Few of the other steady noises to which children are exposed are likely to be present for long-enough periods on a daily basis to pose a significant risk. A clear exception to this general rule occurs among those exposed to loud machinery as a part of daily chores or vocational training. A study of hearing levels in children raised on working farms reported that 15% showed significantly poorer hearing than did age-matched control populations.[8] This hearing loss was seen only among those actively engaged in chores involving noisy machinery. Similar trends may exist among those in vocational training programs such as woodworking and welding.

Factors Influencing Susceptibility to NIHL

Despite much research in this area, a useful predictor of susceptibility to NIHL does not exist. Of special interest in a pediatric context is the large literature suggesting that young individuals are more susceptible to NIHL than are older individuals. Unfortunately, such research has been carried out only in rodents, and we can only speculate as to whether the results are applicable to humans.[9] Nevertheless, the possibility exists that more stringent exposure guidelines for the pediatric population should be developed.

Ear Protection

There are two basic kinds of ear protectors available to consumers today: an earmuff type and an inserted type.[10] Foam inserts are a little trickier to install properly, but many prefer them because, once in place, they are essentially invisible. In a pinch, a ball of (warm) wet cotton may be inserted into the ear canal (dry cotton will accomplish nothing). Both types of ear protectors can provide significant signal attenuation, close to 40 dB in the important midfrequency region, if fitted properly and left undisturbed. Under more realistic conditions (fitted perhaps improperly by a user who then may engage in strenuous physical activity), the maximum attenuations are closer to 20 dB. Nevertheless, even 20 dB of attenuation will reduce many steady-state noise exposures to below the 90-dB(A) line and most impulse noise to below the 140-dB OSHA limit. Thus, if hearing protection is used, it should be possible to maintain a noisy hobby as well as good hearing throughout life.

References

1. Liberman MC, Mulroy MJ: Acute and chronic effects of acoustic trauma: Cochlear pathology and auditory-nerve pathophysiology, in Hamernik RP, Henderson D, Salvi R (eds): *New Perspectives on Noise-Induced Hearing Loss.* New York: Raven Press, 1982, pp 105-135.
2. Passchier-Vermeer W: Hearing loss due to continuous exposure to steady state broadband noise. *J Acoust Soc Am* 1974;56:1585.
3. Hazell J: *Tinnitus.* Edinburgh: Churchill Livingstone, 1987.
4. Taylor GD, Williams E: Acoustic trauma in the sports hunter. *Laryngoscope* 1966;76:863.
5. Gupta D, Vishwakarma MS: Toy weapons and firecrackers: A source of hearing loss. *Laryngoscope* 1989;99:330.
6. Hughes E, Fortnum HM, Davis AC, et al: Damage to hearing arising from leisure noise. *Br J Audiol* 1986;20:157.
7. Catalano PJ, Levin SM: Noise-induced hearing loss and portable radios with headphones. *Int J Pediatr Otorhinolaryngol* 1985;9:59.
8. Broste SK, Hansen DA, Strand RL, et al: Hearing loss among high school farm students. *Am J Public Health* 1989;79:619.
9. Mills JH: Noise and children: A review of literature. *J Acoust Soc Am* 1975;58:767.
10. Alberti PW, Riko K, Abel SM, Kristensen R: The effectiveness of hearing protectors in practice. *J Otolaryngol* 1979;8:354.

Discussion

Dr Luxford: I use tobramycin eyedrops as eardrops all the time for children who have draining ears that are poorly responsive to other forms of medication. At our office, we use chloramphenicol topically for patients who have draining mastoid cavities.

Dr Brookhouser: There is possible synergism between ototoxic drugs and noise. Older children and adolescents who are being treated for tumors with antineoplastic drugs sit around the hospital listening to personal cassette players, to help overcome their boredom. People who are losing their hearing due to noise don't realize what is happening, and they tend to turn the volume up to compensate for it.

Dr Thornton: The effects of noise exposure in an impaired ear are different from those in a normal ear, and the difference is not just a linear cumulation. The permanent threshold shift associated with a given level of noise exposure eventually reaches a plateau, and continued exposure at that level does not keep increasing the hearing loss. I want to be very sure, however, that we don't perpetuate the old adage that an impaired ear is protected against noise. That is not true.

An impaired ear is not necessarily as sensitive to the same levels of noise that would cause damage in a normal-hearing ear. The hearing-aid worry is one that, if misinterpreted, can actually do damage by causing people to have underpowered or underfitted hearing aids.

Dr Grundfast: I want to raise the question of genetic predisposition to or protection from noise-induced trauma. I have heard it suggested that, varying with pigment, there is a variation in susceptibility. That is, brown-eyed individuals with brown hair and melanocytes in the stria vascularis are less sensitive to noise-induced trauma and to the effects of aminoglycosides than are blue-eyed individuals who have prematurely gray hair.

Dr Liberman: My interpretation of the literature on the possible relationship between pigmentation and susceptibility to noise-induced hearing loss is that the effects in many of the human studies are small, certainly with respect to eye color, and sometimes contradictory. In animal studies of pigmented versus albino rodents, where all the variables can be controlled, there is no conclusive evidence for effects of pigmentation on susceptibility to noise.

Dr Grundfast: Albino animals lack melanocytes. Spotting mutant animals—and there are many spotting mutant mice—have melanocytes in certain parts of the body and not in other parts. Some spotting mutant animals are more susceptible to noise-induced hearing loss and also to hearing loss from aminoglycosides.

Dr Bess: Mills wrote a very comprehensive article on noise and children in the 1970s [*J Acoust Soc Am* 1975;58:768], in which he implied that children could be more susceptible than adults to a given noise exposure. I wonder if anyone has ever followed up on that or done any later research in that area.

Is there a greater prevalence of hearing loss in young children as a consequence of the noise exposure that they are receiving today?

Dr Liberman: Noise-damage risk criteria are mainly based on studies of adults and may not be applicable to children. The idea that children are at higher risk is based solely on animal studies. A large number of controlled studies on rodents show that if you take guinea pigs or mice or rats at a very young age, between 0 and 30 days, overexpose them to noise, and compare their hearing loss or ear damage to that of adult animals of the same species, there are major differences. As far as I know, this has never been studied in humans.

Dr Ruben: A study in Scandinavia 7 or 8 years ago [Ruben, *Int J Pediatr Otorhinolaryngol* 1985;9:1] showed a higher incidence of hearing loss in teenagers. Rural youngsters are at risk from guns and snowmobiles.

Dr Harris: General pediatricians provide anticipatory guidance to their patients on common risk situations. Are there guidelines that pediatricians should give to parents, based on what has been said about personal stereos?

Dr Liberman: They should point out the real risk of playing in a rock band, where the potential for noise-induced hearing loss is well documented. As for personal cassette players, the possibility for ear damage clearly exists. Although existing studies suggest that few people listen at high-enough levels for long-enough periods to cause permanent damage, such studies have not assessed very-long-term effects, which may occur over decades.

Dr Harris: So those who play in rock bands should be getting foam?

Dr Liberman: Yes, they should wear foam earplugs.

Dr Klein: They want to hear. They want to come in on the beat.

Dr Liberman: Yes, but foam earplugs will merely attenuate the sound out of the damaging range. It will still be clearly audible.

Dr Eavey: Do any data show the need for legislation to modify the maximum volume of cassette players so that youngsters receive only 80 dB instead of 130 dB?

Dr Liberman: I am not sure that existing data strongly support an urgent need to restrict the maximum output of cassette players. However, I think this would be a highly appropriate area for warning labels.

Dr Brookhouser: It is very difficult to get good data in the United States on the incidence of hearing impairment. I would urge our pediatric colleagues to consider screening children after they get into junior and senior high school, to try to acquire baseline data.

The Armed Services have had to revise their admitting criteria for hearing. To adequately staff the volunteer Army, they allow for the presence of bilateral high-frequency hearing loss. This indicates to me a public health concern, in that a significant number of potential recruits apparently have such impairment.

Dr Klein: Were the same standards used before?

Dr Brookhouser: No. Earlier, they would allow significant loss in one ear, but the other ear had to be normal. Now, they allow for bilateral high-frequency loss.

Session II—
Conductive Hearing Loss: Epidemiology, Etiology, and Pathogenesis

Hearing Loss and Otitis Media: Epidemiology, Etiology, and Pathogenesis
Jerome O. Klein, MD

Points To Recall:
- Risk factors for recurrent and severe acute otitis media (AOM) include male sex, race, first episodes at an early age, sibling history of severe middle ear infections, being bottle fed, and attendance in group day care.
- Middle ear effusion (MEE) persists for weeks to months after every episode of AOM, although appropriate antibiotic therapy sterilizes MEE within a few days. The pathogenesis of persistent MEE is uncertain.
- Conductive hearing loss (median = 25 dB) occurs when MEE is present. Infants with recurrent AOM may be at risk for developmental delay because of prolonged hearing impairment.
- The bacteriology of AOM suggests choice of antimicrobial agents. Pneumococcus, Haemophilus influenzae, and Moraxella catarrhalis are the major bacterial pathogens.

Considerations for Referral:
- Children with severe and recurrent AOM who fail to improve with prophylactic antibiotics should be referred to an otolaryngologist for possible placement of ventilating tubes and/or adenoidectomy.
- Children with prolonged MEE (more than 3 months) should be referred to an otolaryngologist for evaluation. The referral should be considered earlier if there is a history of impairment of hearing.
- Children with recurrent AOM who have other focal infections (eg, pneumonia, suppurative skin and soft-tissue infections, or adenitis) should be referred to an immunologist because of concern for underlying disease affecting the immune system.

Acute otitis media and middle ear effusion are among the most common illnesses of childhood. After every episode of AOM, fluid persists in the middle ear for varying periods, usually weeks to months. The signs of acute infection resolve with appropriate antibiotic therapy, but the MEE, now sterile (in episodes of bacterial infection), persists. The type of antibiotic—β-lactam, macrolide, or sulfonamide—does not appear to influence the duration of MEE.

Conductive hearing loss usually accompanies MEE, although the extent of the loss varies from child to child. Because of the frequency of AOM and accompanying hearing loss, pediatricians have been concerned that children who suffer from persisting or recurrent middle ear disease might also suffer from delay or impairment of speech, language, or cognitive abilities (Figure).

HEARING LOSS ASSOCIATED WITH MIDDLE EAR EFFUSION

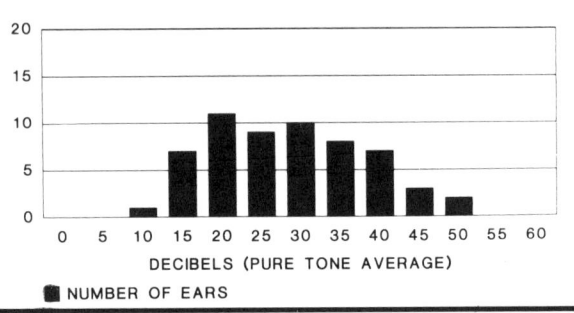

[bar chart: NUMBER OF EARS vs DECIBELS (PURE TONE AVERAGE), values 0 to 60]

Figure. Evaluation of children before placement of ventilating tubes.[1]

To prevent the conductive hearing loss associated with otitis media, we need to identify the characteristics of the children at risk and prevent or aggressively manage their disease to minimize the time spent with MEE. There are many studies of the epidemiology and microbiology of otitis media, but there are scant data about the pathogenesis of MEE.

Definitions

For the purposes of discussion, AOM is defined as effusion in one or both middle ears accompanied by one or more signs of acute illness, including earache, otorrhea, ear tugging, fever, irritability, lethargy, anorexia, vomiting, or diarrhea. MEE is the presence of liquid in one or both ears.

Conductive Hearing Loss and Otitis Media

Audiograms of children with MEE usually indicate a mild to moderate conductive hearing loss. The median loss is approximately 25 dB.[1] Conductive hearing loss due to the presence of MEE appears to be influenced less by the quality of the fluid (serous, mucoid, or purulent) than by the volume (partially or completely filling the middle ear space). The conductive hearing impairment is usually reversed with resolution of the MEE. In the absence of MEE, high negative pressure in the middle ear or atelectasis may also result in conductive hearing loss.

Few studies of hearing have been performed during episodes of AOM. Olmstead and co-workers[2] in 1964 documented moderate hearing loss in children during the period immediately after the acute episode and throughout a 6-month period of observation. To my knowledge, no other audiologic studies have been performed during AOM. Our concern for hearing loss during and following the acute infection is based on data developed in audiologic studies of children with MEE of long duration. The dynamics of hearing loss during acute infections may be different, and more data are needed to clarify the course of hearing loss at the onset of AOM and during the period of persistent MEE that follows the acute infection.

Sensorineural Hearing Loss and Otitis Media

Sensorineural hearing loss is uncommonly associated with AOM. A permanent sensorineural loss has been described, presumably as a result of spread of microorganisms or products of inflammation through the round window membrane or due to a suppurative complication of AOM such as labyrinthitis. Permanent hearing loss may also result from irreversible inflammatory changes such as those that result from adhesive otitis media or ossicular discontinuity.

Epidemiology

Otitis media is a disease of infants and young children. By 3 years of age, most children have had at least one episode of AOM and as many as 50% of children have had recurrent AOM (three or more episodes). The peak age-specific attack rate occurs during the second half of the 1st year of life. Few children have first episodes of AOM after 3 years of age.[3]

Among the variables that are associated with AOM are 1) sex (males have more middle ear disease than females), 2) race (there is an extraordinary incidence of infection in some racial groups such as Native Americans, Alaskan and Canadian Eskimos, and African and Australian aboriginal children), 3) age at first episode (the earlier in life the first episode occurs, the more likely the child is to have recurrent disease), 4) sibling history of AOM and recurrent AOM (suggesting a genetic basis for the disease), 5) bottle feeding (infants who are breastfed for as short a period as 3 months have less AOM in the 1st year of life than do children who are not breastfed), and 6) frequent exposure to infectious agents, such as occurs in day-care centers.[3,4]

Age at first episode of AOM has been demonstrated to be an important predictor of recurrent AOM in many studies. These data suggest that an early episode of AOM is a marker for special susceptibility to ear infections and that the children may have an underlying predisposition that may be based on anatomic, physiologic, or immunologic factors. This concept is supported by the correlation of AOM in the index case and history of ear disease in siblings. These data support a genetic basis for severe and recurrent disease.

Few interracial studies have been done, and therefore we cannot fully evaluate the significance of the extent and severity of ear disease in different racial groups. Poverty, extremes of climate (temperature, humidity, altitude), crowding in the home, inadequate hygiene, poor sanitation, and lack of medical care are still to be explored as factors in the high incidence of disease in some racial groups.

Breastfed infants were shown to be at lower risk for AOM than infants who were exclusively bottle fed.[3] The association did not increase with increased duration of breastfeeding. The mechanism for the protective effect of breast milk or a harmful effect of cow's milk or infant formula is not known. The hypothesis that breast milk is protective is substantiated by studies of a special feeding bottle for infants with cleft palate. Infants who were fed with a bottle containing breast milk had fewer days of MEE than did infants who were fed with the device containing formula, suggesting that protection was more likely due to a constituent in breast milk rather than to the mode of feeding.

Passive smoking may affect pulmonary function in children, but data are less clear about an effect of exposure to cigarette smoking in the household and disease of the middle ear in children. Objective information about exposure and data about duration and intensity of smoke in the environment are needed to clarify the association between cigarette smoking and otitis media.

Etiology and Pathogenesis of AOM

The development of otitis media is best explained by the following sequence of events: 1) a microbial or environmental event causes congestion of the mucous membrane of the upper respiratory tract; the congestion includes the nasopharynx, eustachian tube, and middle ear; 2) congestion of the mucosa in the eustachian tube results in obstruction of the narrowest portion of the tube, the isthmus; 3) secretions of the mucous membrane of the middle ear accumulate behind the eustachian tube obstruction; 4) microbial pathogens are constantly washed in and out of the middle ear, but with obstruction of the eustachian tube the organisms have no egress and multiply, resulting in an acute infection.

For some children with severe and recurrent episodes of otitis media, there is an underlying anatomic (eg, cleft palate), immunologic (eg, chronic granulomatous disease), or physiologic (eg, eustachian tube disability) defect. The vast majority of children, however, have no defined deficit.

The microbiology of AOM has been documented by cultures of MEE. The results of bacterial studies from the United States, western Europe, Japan, and Central and South America have been remarkably consistent from place to place and from time to time: Pneumococcus is cultured from approximately one third of cases of AOM; *Haemophilus influenzae* (nontypable) is isolated from about 20% to 30%; *Moraxella catarrhalis* is obtained from 7% to 20% of middle ear fluids; and a small number of cases are associated with gram-negative enteric bacilli, *Staphylococcus aureus*, and group A streptococci. Approximately one third of MEEs do not have a bacterial pathogen. Respiratory viruses, including respiratory syncytial virus, influenza, adenoviruses, and rhinoviruses, have been isolated alone or concurrently with bacteria.

Chlamydia has been isolated from infants, and mycoplasma infections in school-age children have been associated with otitis media.

Etiology and Pathogenesis of Persistent MEE

The reason(s) for prolonged duration of MEE after episodes of AOM is still uncertain. The appropriate antibacterial agent eradicates the MEE, but the fluid, now sterile, persists. The most likely explanation appears to be a persistent inflammatory reaction due, perhaps, to microbiologic antigens that persist after the organisms have been eradicated. Rational management of persistent MEE must await clarification of the etiology and pathogenesis.

References
1. Fria TJ, Cantekin EI, Eichler JA: Hearing acuity of children with otitis media with effusion. *Arch Otolaryngol* 1985;111:10.
2. Olmstead RW, Alvarez MC, Moroney JD, Eversden M: The pattern of hearing following acute otitis media. *J Pediatr* 1964;65:252.
3. Teele DW, Klein JO, Rosner B, and Greater Boston Otitis Media Study Group: Epidemiology of otitis media during the first seven years of life in children in greater Boston: A prospective, cohort study. *J Infect Dis* 1989;160:83.
4. Wald ER, Dashefsky B, Byers C, et al: Frequency and severity of infections in day care. *J Pediatr* 1988;112:540.

Structural Reasons for Conductive Hearing Loss
Roland D. Eavey, MD

Points To Recall:
- *An abnormal appearance of the auricle, canal, or middle ear can alert the clinician to a possible hearing loss.*
- *To check for a possible hearing loss, there is no substitute for a hearing test.*
- *A conductive hearing loss often can be surgically corrected.*

Considerations for Referral:
- *An abnormal-appearing auricle*
- *Skin tags*
- *A narrow ear canal*
- *A polyp or mass in the ear canal*
- *A foreign body that cannot be easily removed*
- *Tympanic membrane perforation*
- *Persistent otorrhea*

- Cholesteatoma
- A mass in the middle ear
- Evidence of abnormal ossicles
- A conductive hearing loss without obvious cause

There are many mechanical reasons that sound may fail to conduct through the external and middle ear to the inner ear. A conductive type of loss usually is, at maximum, approximately 60 dB, corresponding to a residual "bottom half" of hearing ability. If a conductive loss is superimposed on an existing sensorineural loss, the total deficit will be additive.

The patient with a conductive hearing loss has two main advantages compared to a patient with sensorineural hearing loss. First, the reason for a loss can often be seen otoscopically, which will alert the pediatrician to further evaluate the situation by hearing testing. Second, the condition and the hearing frequently can be surgically corrected or else the hearing can be satisfactorily amplified with a hearing aid.

External Ear

Congenital malformation of the auricle (microtia) and external ear canal (aural atresia) is a rare but easily understood reason for a conductive hearing loss. The auricle is malformed and usually no meatus or canal is present. The incidence is approximately 1 in 10,000 children. Unilateral cases are more common than bilateral cases.[1] The etiology can be known with certainty only in cases of either vitamin A embryonic teratogenicity[2] or intrauterine deformation. However, animal models demonstrate that this malformation may develop either from rupture of the embryonic stapedial artery or from failure of neural-crest migration.[3,4]

The pediatrician should be able to provide assistance in several ways: First, a hearing test must be obtained. In the newborn, a brain-stem evoked-response hearing test is necessary. Second, counsel can be provided to the parents that the external auricular malformation can be corrected. The hearing also can be corrected in selected cases. Third, if the microtia is bilateral, amplification by a bone-conduction hearing aid should be used. Fourth, in unilateral cases, the pediatrician should conduct routine otoscopic surveillance to make sure that the "normal" ear does not develop otitis media with effusion that will then create a bilateral hearing loss. Fifth, since the ear with the atresia still can develop acute otitis media, suspected ear infections should be treated. Mastoiditis has been reported in aural atresia.[5]

Surgical correction of microtia starts with auricular reconstruction at about 6 years of age. Carved rib and soft-tissue transposition are used to create an ear with a realistic appearance (Fig 1). If the congenital middle ear malformation shown by computed tomography is not severe, the patient theoretically may be operable for hearing reconstruction after auricular reconstruction has been initiated.

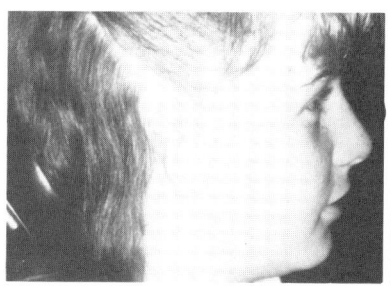

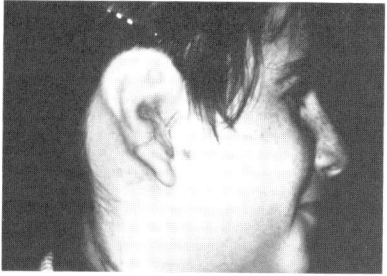

Fig 1. *Left*: An adolescent with a typical right-sided congenital microtia and skin tag. *Right*: Shortly after surgical correction by author.

A more common external congenital abnormality is the skin tag. This condition tends to be trivialized, and some physicians will even tie a loop around the base so that the tag will amputate. However, this tag can signal other anomalies in the middle ear that might not be obvious with otoscopy. Therefore, a hearing test is prudent, since one patient with a skin tag may have normal hearing but another may have a 60-dB hearing loss. Further, a preferred removal treatment for skin tags is surgical excision with cosmetic closure that eliminates the subcutaneous cartilaginous mound that persists when the base has been tied.

External Auditory Canal

Canal stenosis is another congenital reason for impaired sound conduction. This malformation occurs because the final stage of embryonic ear formation, mesenchymal resorption between the meatus and the middle ear, has failed to occur fully. The incidence of canal stenosis is not known. Often the auricle is normally formed so that delay in diagnosis is often several years.[6] Besides the conductive hearing loss that will occur, the patient is at some risk of developing a cholesteatoma. With a pinhole-sized canal, the likelihood of developing a cholesteatoma during childhood is greater than 90% by 12 years of age.[7] If drainage occurs in a stenotic ear canal or if squamous material or a polyp is seen, referral to an otolaryngologist is mandatory.

The treatment for a narrow external auditory canal can be watchful waiting if the child actually has good hearing in the other ear. However, if bilateral malformation or cholesteatoma is present, then an operative procedure can be performed. A new eardrum can be placed and the ossicles evaluated and repaired at the time of surgery. Fig 2 shows the preoperative and postoperative audiograms of a patient who had canal stenosis and cholesteatoma.

Other reasons exist for a conductive hearing loss in the normally formed ear canal. The most obvious reason would be cerumen impaction. While it is true that many children have sufficient cerumen to

AUDIOGRAM
Frequency (Hz)

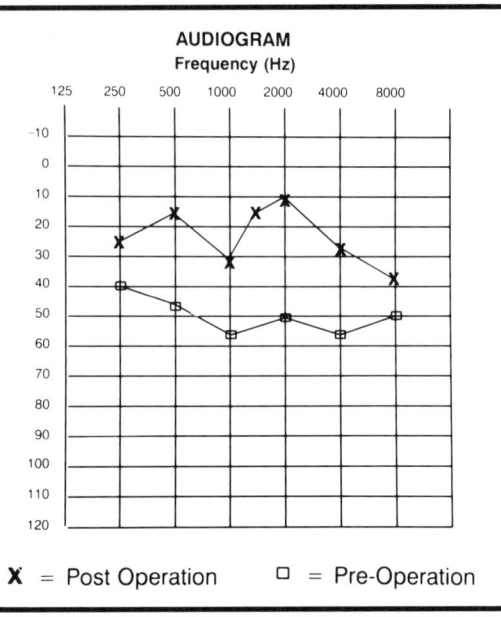

Fig 2. An audiogram of a 10-year-old boy with a left-sided canal stenosis and conductive loss (□ - □ - □). The ear was surgically improved, providing him a disease-free, dry, open canal and a hearing gain (✕ - ✕ - ✕).

obscure the view of the tympanic membrane, to the frustration of many health care providers, it is the rare child who actually presents with a hearing loss exclusively due to wax. However, a generous impaction can cause a hearing loss of about 30 dB.

A foreign body in the external auditory canal can also cause a conductive hearing loss. Not only does the foreign body occlude the canal, but often the irritation produces canal-skin edema that further blocks sound conduction.

External otitis can also be associated with a conductive hearing loss if severe. In this case, the patient usually has an exquisitely painful canal and tragus. Other conditions can appear otoscopically exactly like an external otitis, such as acute mastoiditis and eosinophilic granuloma of the temporal bone, which can break through the bone cortex and cause the canal to narrow. The hearing will demonstrate a conductive loss until the canal regains patency.

A mass, such as an aural polyp, can be present in the external auditory canal. An aural polyp can signal very rare disorders, such as rhabdomyosarcoma or eosinophilic granuloma, but is most often seen as part of an inflammatory response to keratinized squamous epithelium. This granulation tissue can be noted in the presence of a ventilation tube. This is not a reaction to the tube. Instead, the squamous epithelium of the lateral surface of the drum and the middle ear mucosal surface of the drum come into contact and an inflammatory response is incited.

Similar-appearing granulation tissue will develop in response to the keratinized squamous epithelium of a cholesteatoma.

Tympanic Membrane

A common cause of conductive hearing loss would be a large perforation, usually the result of chronic ear disease. Interestingly, a small perforation probably does little harm. In fact, one can reflect on the fact that a ventilation tube maintains a small perforation and usually is associated with hearing gain. However, the larger the perforation, the smaller the surface area of the tympanic membrane to capture sound. Additional damage to the ossicles may be associated with a large perforation.

The tympanic membrane may also be abnormal due to tympanosclerosis that can occur after either spontaneous drum rupture or myringotomy. Fortunately, tympanosclerosis usually is not associated with hearing loss even if the drum appears to be almost entirely snow-white. But a thick plaque, especially if associated with tympanosclerosis of the middle ear space, may be too stiff to transmit sound effectively. The tympanic membrane, conversely, may be very thin and retracted and fail to transmit sound effectively (Fig 3).

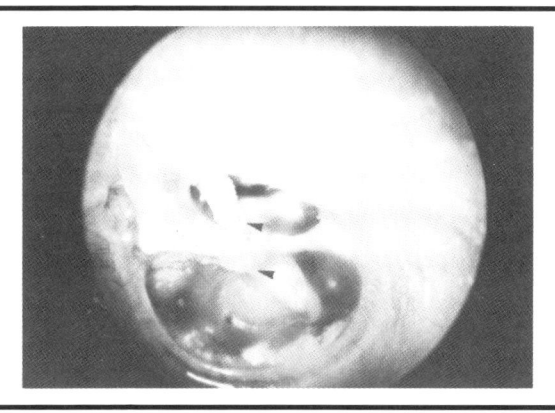

Fig 3. A severely retracted tympanic membrane draped over the ossicles. Upper arrow is the incudostapedial joint; lower arrow is the point of contact of the retracted malleus onto the promontory.

Ossicles

Congenital ossicular anomalies can be present even if no obvious otoscopic abnormality can be appreciated. Conditions such as malleus fixation or stapes fixation may be present. The malleus fixes superiorly above the view permitted by the tympanic membrane.[8] The stapes fixes in the oval window niche. Treatment for these conditions is either surgery or hearing amplification. The goals for the pediatrician are to identify the hearing loss and then to refer the child for evaluation and treatment. Timing of the surgery may depend on the child's coincidental propensity to develop otitis media with effusion.

Stapedial fixation also occurs due to otosclerosis. However, this diagnosis is much more common in adults than in children. Bone diseases such as osteogenesis imperfecta can also cause overgrowth at the stapes/oval window interface. Any abnormality of the size or shape of the malleus, incus, and stapes or any condition that makes ossicular motion either too flaccid or too rigid will impede optimal conduction of sound and diminish hearing. For example, ossicular damage can occur from chronic otitis media and from trauma.

Often the audiologist or otolaryngologist is not absolutely certain of the particular ossicular abnormality that may be present in a patient who has a conductive hearing loss in the absence of otitis media with effusion. The best way to evaluate this is to surgically explore the ear. This permits the ossicles to be viewed and palpated to ascertain the best method of correction. If surgery either is not possible or should fail to provide improvement in hearing, a hearing aid is an excellent alternative.

Middle Ear Space

The middle ear space may also contain material that interferes with the conduction of sound. The most common reason would obviously be otitis media with effusion.

Cholesteatoma is a destructive middle ear process that occurs in approximately 5 patients per 100,000 population.[9,10] Various theories are used to explain how keratinized squamous epithelial cells might be located in the middle ear. Some patients are noted to have a white pearl behind a normal tympanic membrane, as if embryonic rest cells had grown[11] or amniotic fluid cellular elements had proliferated.[12] Other theories of cholesteatoma involve changes in the tympanic membrane, such as from retraction or perforation. The keratinized squamous epithelial cells proliferate and damage the ossicles, the tympanic membrane, and any bone covering the brain, facial nerve, or inner ear. Damage is believed to be due both to enzymatic destruction[13] and to pressure exerted by the expanding mass.[14] This tissue frequently incites an inflammatory response and polyp formation. It can become infected and associated with otorrhea. Treatment for cholesteatoma is complete surgical removal.

Other situations exist in which foreign material is present in the ear. Even after birth, mesenchyme can occasionally still be found in the middle ear. The amount of mesenchyme varies from nonexistent to enough to nearly fill the middle ear space. Temporal bone histologic analysis also reveals that it is common for the infant middle ear space to contain amniotic fluid cellular contents such as squamous cells and even hair. In neonates, the incidence is about 90%.[12] The size of the inoculum can vary from a trace to enough to fill a substantial portion of the middle ear cleft.[15] The cellular content initiates an intense inflammatory response, producing granulation tissue and adhesion (Fig 4). Additionally, the child theoretically could become otitis-media-prone due to this inflammation, which would then set up a cycle that would continue conductive hearing loss.

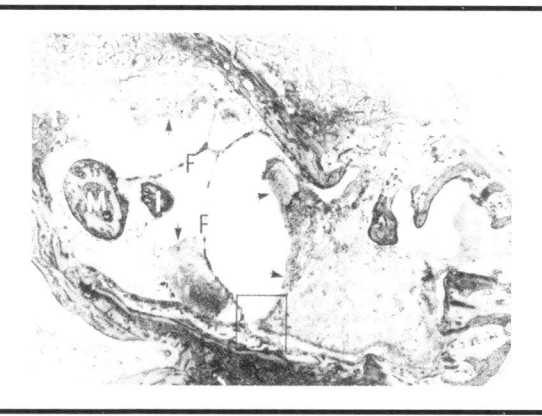

Fig 4. Histopathologic section of an infant's temporal bone demonstrating amniotic fluid cellular contents inciting a reaction of granulation tissue.[12] M = malleus, I = incus, F = mucosal folds, arrows = granulation tissue. Box around an attachment area from mucosa to granulation tissue. Reprinted with permission.

Blood can enter the middle ear space. In newborns, this is noted to correlate with bloody amniotic fluid. In older children, it would occur after head trauma or from a condition such as leukemia. Blood will cause a substantial conductive hearing loss and usually takes about 2 to 4 weeks for clearance. An audiogram is necessary, even after the blood is no longer otoscopically visible, to assess auditory acuity, especially after trauma.

Osteoma, a benign bone growth, can be present in the middle ear, causing hearing loss. An osteoma tends to be round and white and must be distinguished from cholesteatoma. Treatment is surgical.

The primary-care physician is the child's first and best ally in regard to ear disease. Many of the reasons for conductive hearing loss are visible. Many of the conditions can be favorably treated by surgery or a hearing aid. Although otitis media with effusion is by far the most common cause of conductive loss, other conditions should also be kept in mind so that we can offer our patients healthy hearing.

References

1. Eavey RD: Management of congenital ear malformations, in Grundfast K (ed): *Pediatr Clin North Am* 1989;36:1521.
2. Lemmer E, Chen D, Hoar R, et al: Retinoic acid embryopathy. *N Engl J Med* 1985;313:837.
3. Phelps P, Poswillo D, Lloyd G: The ear deformities in mandibulofacial dysostosis (Treacher Collins syndrome). *Clin Otolaryngol* 1981;6:15.

4. Poswillo D: The pathogenesis of the first and second branchial arch syndrome. *Oral Surg* 1973;35:302.
5. Zalzal GH: Acute mastoiditis complicated by sigmoid sinus thrombosis in congenital aural atresia. *Int J Pediatr Otorhinolaryngol* 1987;14:31.
6. Grundfast KM, Camilon F: External auditory canal stenosis and partial atresia without associated anomalies. *Ann Otol Rhinol Laryngol* 1986;95:505.
7. Cole RR, Jahrsdoerfer RA: The risk of cholesteatoma in congenital aural stenosis. *Laryngoscope* 1990;100:576.
8. Schuknecht HF: *Pathology of the Ear*. Cambridge, Mass: Harvard University Press, 1974, p 188.
9. Ruben RJ: The disease in society: Evaluation of chronic otitis media in general and cholesteatoma in particular, in Sade J (ed): *Cholesteatoma and Mastoid Surgery*, Proceedings of the Second International Conference on Cholesteatoma. Amsterdam: Kugler Publications, 1982, pp 111-116.
10. Dominguez S, Harker LA: Incidence of cholesteatoma with cleft palate. *Ann Otol Rhinol Laryngol* 1988;97:659.
11. Levenson MJ, Michaels L, Parisier SC, Juarbe C: Congenital cholesteatomas in children: An embryologic correlation. *Laryngoscope* 1988;98:949.
12. Northrup C, Piza J, Eavey R: Histological observations of amniotic fluid cellular contents in the ears of neonates and infants. *Int J Pediatr Otolaryngol* 1986;11:113.
13. Abramson M, Huang CC: Localization of collagenase in human middle ear cholesteatoma. *Laryngoscope* 1977;87:771.
14. Drissek BS, Chole RA: Pressures exerted by experimental cholesteatomas. *Arch Otolaryngol Head Neck Surg* 1987;113:386.
15. Piza J, Gonzalez M, Northrup C, Eavey R: Meconium contamination of the neonatal middle ear. *J Pediatr* 1989;115:910.

Discussion

Dr Thornton: From a practical standpoint for pediatricians, mild conductive hearing loss often masks identification of a mild sensorineural loss. The hearing loss in a child who has a fluctuating 10- to 20-dB hearing loss often goes unnoticed by the parents. But with a 30-dB sensorineural hearing loss, that 10- to 20-dB conductive overlay drops the hearing to a level where the loss becomes quite noticeable. The parents get concerned and bring the child in.

What often happens is that the physician looks in the ear, sees an explanation for the decreased hearing, does not get a hearing test, treats the child, and the hearing improves 10 to 20 dB until another episode of otitis media occurs. These are the children that you pick up in school at the age of 6 or 7 years, who have never had a hearing test but who have had recurrent otitis media. This is why it is worthwhile to administer a hearing test with each occurrence of otitis media.

Dr Grundfast: For many years, we have talked about the sequelae of otitis media in terms of hearing impairment. But what concerns me is that some children who have had otitis media, whether or not they have had tympanostomy tubes in their ears, develop a retraction pocket in the posterior-superior portion of the eardrum.

It often starts with the eardrum resting on the lenticular process of the incus. This is easily observable by most pediatricians and family practitioners using a pneumatic otoscope. It occurs usually between the ages of 3 and 7 years, and if it progresses, it leads to erosion of the lenticular process of the incus and to the need for surgery. If the retraction pocket has a narrow neck, it leads to the development of cholesteatoma, which can progress into the area called the facial recess or the sinus tympani, from which it is extremely difficult to remove.

Patients who have this disorder, which can range from a minor to a serious problem, often wind up with conductive hearing loss, which is permanent. If they have reconstructive surgery and the ossicular chain is restored to continuity, hearing in the range of 20- to 25-dB thresholds can sometimes be restored. But the many children who go on to develop cholesteatoma wind up with 40- or 50-dB thresholds after one or more operative procedures.

Pediatricians can help us by looking carefully for this condition, and otologists can deal with it by operating earlier than we have been.

Dr Combs: Are the ears of normal full-term infants ventilated at the same time as the lungs?

Dr Klein: We have been examining infants otoscopically in our NICU. During the first 24 hours of life, the canal is filled with vernix, and examination of the tympanic membrane is often difficult. After the first 24 hours, the examination is almost easier than in older children, because the external ear canal is shorter. Because of the short eustachian tube, we often see movement with breathing. The vast majority of infants within the select population of the NICU have ventilated ears at first examination or by the end of the 1st day of life.

Dr Combs: Might there be a small subset of otitis-prone infants whose ears are ventilated at a later date? There may be a small subset of infants who have effusion that persists during the first 2 months of life and who are then otitis-prone.

Dr Eavey: I don't believe that ears of newborn infants look normal for several weeks. The majority will not look "normal" compared to those of a 3-month-old that are "normal." But normality at 1 week is different from normality at 3 months. Blood, pus, or amber effusions will be seen in the middle ear, just as in an older child with a chronic effusion. You cannot see mesenchyme, but you can see a thickened drum that doesn't seem to move very well, and you can infer that something is going on behind the drum.

Dr Klein: We see many infants born to mothers who are addicted to intravenous drugs. Often these infants have thick and less-mobile drums. They also have congestion of the upper respiratory tract, and otoscopic observations are consistent with congestion throughout the respiratory mucosa. During our year of observation, the children born to addicted mothers did not have a higher incidence of later otitis media. Whatever the tympanic membrane observations in the newborn period, the changes did not have functional significance later in infancy [Word B, Klein J, unpublished data].

Dr Bess: We have examined 80 or 90 children with unilateral sensorineural hearing loss of 45 dB or greater in the impaired ear, and have found that about 50% of these children have either failed a grade or need resource assistance in school. Children with unilateral loss are at 10 times greater risk for academic failure than are children with normal hearing. Subjects with right-ear impairment are at five times greater risk than subjects with left-ear impairment. Unilateral hearing loss can indeed result in psychoeducational complications.

Dr Eavey: Does it make a difference whether the loss is conductive or sensorineural?

Dr Bess: We followed only sensorineural hearing-impaired subjects. However, I would be concerned about children who have losses of 45 or 50 dB or more, even if they are conductive.

Session III— Hearing Testing

Audiometry Primer

Barbara S. Herrmann, PhD

Points To Recall:
- *Reliable hearing tests are possible for children of any age, including neonates.*
- *A child whose hearing is questioned for any reason should have a hearing test.*
- *The basic measures of hearing tests are similar for all ages; the type of patient response changes with age.*

Considerations for Referral:
- *The question of hearing is raised for any reason, by the parent or any person in contact with the child*
- *Any delay in speech or language development*
- *Repeated episodes of otitis media*
- *Failed hearing screening*
- *Risk factors for hearing loss such as noted in **Appendix A***
- *Trouble in school, either academic or behavioral*

The purpose of audiometry is to measure how a person hears. It is especially important to measure the hearing of children, because they are using their hearing to learn in an auditory world. Infants are learning speech and language and older children are absorbing knowledge needed to become contributing members of society. Since hearing loss is an invisible handicap, hearing-impaired behaviors are easily interpreted as personality, behavioral, or mental problems. These misconceptions can be prevented by prompt and accurate diagnosis of hearing loss.

Basic Measures in Audiometry

Hearing Sensitivity for Pure Tones

Central to the assessment of hearing is measuring a patient's threshold for tones of different frequencies. These thresholds represent the softest sound a patient can hear approximately 50% of the time. They are plotted on an audiogram (Figure), which is a graph of hearing levels with sound pressures in decibels (dB HL) versus frequency in hertz (Hz). The aspect ratio of an audiogram and the calibration of audiometers in dB HL are standardized by the American National Standards Institute and should be the same from clinic to clinic. While the frequency range of human hearing is much wider than that measured on the audiogram, typically 20 to 20,000 Hz, the most sensitive part of that range and the area most important for assessing communication handicap is the 250- to 8000-Hz range on the audiogram. The reference of hearing level is the mean hearing for normal, otologically healthy young adults. A whisper is about 20 dB HL, whereas conversational speech is about 60 dB HL. A jet engine would register about 120 dB HL. A threshold in dB HL is the number of decibels an individual's threshold differs from the mean of normal hearing. A threshold of 40 dB HL means that a patient's hearing sensitivity for a particular frequency is 40 dB poorer than normal.

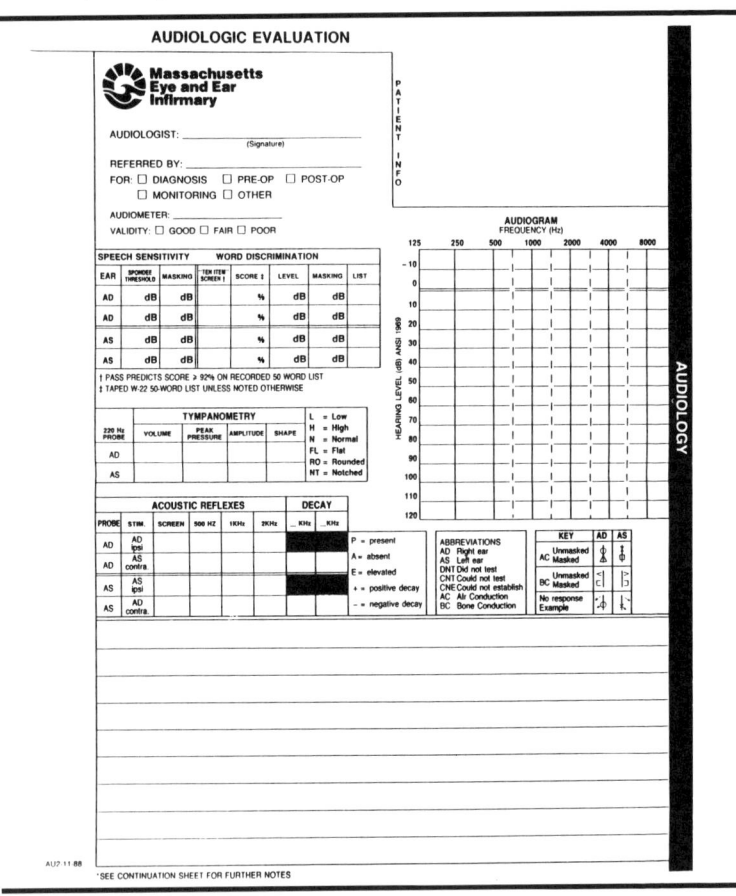

Figure. An audiogram.

In a typical hearing test, thresholds are measured for sounds delivered to the ear in one of two ways, by air conduction or by bone conduction. Air-conduction measurements are those in which the sound travels to the ear via the air. The most familiar of the air-conduction measurements are those made with earphones that measure each ear separately. Air-conduction thresholds can also be measured with a speaker, in which case the hearing of the better ear is tested, since both are available to respond. Air-conduction measurements test the integrity of the entire ear—the outer, middle, and inner ears.

In contrast, bone conduction delivers sound via vibration of the skull, primarily reflecting the integrity of the inner ear. The symbols for air- and bone-conduction thresholds are found in the legend accompanying the audiogram (Figure). Masked thresholds are those obtained with noise in the nontest ear to ensure that the appropriate ear is responding.

The difference between air- and bone-conduction thresholds classifies the type of hearing loss. When air-conduction and bone-conduction thresholds are within ± 5 dB of each other, the site of lesion is the inner ear since the inclusion of the middle and outer ears in air-conduction testing does not change the hearing loss. This type of hearing loss is referred to as sensorineural. Conductive hearing loss means that the bone-conduction thresholds indicate better hearing sensitivity than air-conduction thresholds, indicating problems in the outer or middle ear. The combination of conductive hearing loss and sensorineural hearing loss in the same ear is referred to as a mixed hearing loss.

The degree of hearing loss is classified by the thresholds for each ear. Terms to classify hearing loss are not standardized but are similar across clinics. Commonly used terms and their corresponding threshold ranges are listed in Table 1. For example, a child with moderate hearing loss hears loud speech and develops some speech, albeit impaired, on his or her own. A severely impaired child, on the other hand, develops much less speech and language without help. The profoundly impaired child, who corresponds to most people's conception of a "deaf" child, develops little to no speech and language without rehabilitation. Things become a bit more complicated when the amount of hearing loss is not the same for all frequencies. Hearing losses that occur only for the high frequencies are quite handicapping, and yet, because of the normal hearing sensitivity for some frequencies, the child can hear a pin drop. It is the *distortion* caused by these types of losses that is the primary handicapping factor. The child can hear that something has been said but is unable to distinguish the speech sounds clearly enough to understand.

Table 1. Classification of Hearing Loss.

Hearing Threshold (dB HL) (American National Standards Institute, 1969)	Classification
− 10 to 15	Normal hearing
16 to 25	Slight hearing loss
26 to 40	Mild hearing loss
41 to 55	Moderate hearing loss
56 to 70	Moderately severe hearing loss
70 to 90	Severe hearing loss
90 +	Profound hearing loss

Speech Testing

There are two basic measures of speech in audiometry: 1) the threshold, or level where a person begins to understand or detect speech, and 2) the ability of a patient to understand moderately loud speech. The threshold for speech is frequently used in young children because they tend to respond better to speech than to tones. The threshold for speech by itself, however, has severe limitations. Because speech is a complex acoustic signal containing many frequencies, its threshold represents the best hearing in the ear under test. For example, a patient with a high-frequency hearing loss will have a normal speech threshold because of the normal hearing sensitivity for the low frequencies.

The second speech measure is speech discrimination, or how well someone understands speech when it is loud enough to hear. This test addresses the distortion handicap of hearing loss rather than sensitivity. In adults and older children, the test is most commonly done by using the repetition of single words. This test is done on a limited basis with younger children.

Effect of Age on Testing Techniques

Although the age of a child may greatly affect the method of testing hearing, the goal of defining the hearing sensitivity across the frequency range remains the same. Primarily, only the type of patient response to sound changes with the age of the child (Table 2). Accurate clinical judgments regarding the type of testing method used, the reliability of responses, and the validity of test results are crucial to the successful assessment of hearing in young children. These judgments are best made by an experienced pediatric audiologist.

Table 2. Approximate Age Ranges for Audiometric Testing Procedures.

Patient Age	Testing Procedure
Newborn to 6 months	Evoked-response audiometry (auditory brain-stem response)
6 months to 2½ years	Visual-reinforcement audiometry
2½ years to 4 years	Play audiometry
4 years and older	Adult audiometry

At 4 to 5 years of age, children are frequently as reliable as adults and will raise their hands when a sound is presented. Between the ages of 2½ and 4 years, play audiometry is used, in which a conditioned response, such as putting a peg into a pegboard or dropping blocks into a bucket, is substituted for the hand raise. In many cases, a complete audiogram with bone conduction can be obtained. From the ages of 6 months to about 2 years, a head turn to sound is conditioned by visually reinforcing this response with a lighted toy in a procedure referred to as visual-reinforcement audiometry (VRA). As can be expected, a young child frequently will give reliable responses for only about 20 minutes. During that time, though, a skilled clinician can obtain important thresholds for each ear and sometimes one or two thresholds for bone conduction. If a child will not wear earphones, thresholds are often obtained with a speaker. Results then represent the hearing in the better ear.

There are no reliable behavioral tests of hearing sensitivity for infants younger than 6 months of age. At this age, and in any case where behavioral test results are questioned, it is appropriate to use the auditory brain-stem response, often referred to as ABR or BSER, to measure hearing sensitivity. As with behavioral audiometry, the quality of ABR testing is highly dependent on the technique of the clinicians conducting the test. When done correctly, ABR testing is very accurate and can be done on infants as young as 30 weeks' gestation.[1,2] Using ABR to measure hearing-threshold sensitivity is different from using it to assess neurologic problems. Most clinics only obtain ABR thresholds to clicks. Since clicks are broad-band signals, like speech, their thresholds reflect the best hearing in an ear. It is more desirable to obtain thresholds to frequency-limited signals called tone bursts that can be used to estimate thresholds for different frequencies and, consequently, define hearing sensitivity by frequency.

Unlike the hand raise, which takes about a second, measuring the ABR for a sound near threshold takes about 2 to 5 minutes under good testing conditions. This means that even in a long test session, fewer thresholds can be obtained than for the behavioral tonal audiogram. In our clinic, we routinely obtain thresholds for three frequencies for each ear plus one for bone conduction during a 2-hour test. Testing time is limited because accurate tests cannot be obtained unless a child is sleeping very quietly. In most instances, chloral hydrate is used to ensure an adequate testing state.

Since the amount of information that can be obtained in young children with behavioral or evoked-response audiometry is often limited, a skilled, experienced audiologist is crucial. Confronted with a limited time frame, an astute audiologist will obtain the most important information first. For example, ruling out a handicapping hearing loss is frequently the major concern when testing a young child. Since the threshold at 2000 Hz can determine whether a hearing aid is needed, this threshold is often obtained first. Proper management can still be initiated even if no additional thresholds can be obtained.

Role of Tympanometry

Tympanometry is one of several tests of acoustic impedance used in audiometric testing and is extremely helpful in identifying middle ear disease. The tympanogram is a graph of the mobility of the middle ear mechanism across a range of ear canal pressures. Physical changes in the middle ear structures, such as middle ear fluid or disarticulation of the ossicles, are reflected by the amplitude and shape of the tympanogram.

Flat tympanograms or those with low amplitude indicate stiff middle ear mechanisms, such as those caused by otitis media or ossicular fixation. Notched tympanograms or those with large amplitude are indicative of highly mobile middle ears, such as those with ossicular discontinuities. The pressure corresponding to the greatest mobility of the middle ear is also useful to document changes in middle ear pressure.

Tympanometry in an audiologic setting is usually done when a conductive component is present. Another application, well suited to the pediatrician's office, is using tympanometry in conjunction with a medical examination to help identify middle ear disease and to monitor children during treatment. Children with repeated middle ear disease can be flagged for hearing-test referral. Other tests of acoustic impedance, such as acoustic reflex testing or eustachian tube testing, are better used in conjunction with other tests in the otolaryngologic and audiologic settings.

The relation of tympanometry to hearing sensitivity is often confused. Tympanometry does not measure hearing sensitivity. One can have normal tympanograms and a significant sensorineural loss. On the other hand, a patient can have abnormal tympanograms and still have hearing within normal limits. Even more complex is the child who has middle ear disease that can be nicely tracked by tympanometry but who also has an underlying sensorineural hearing loss. Hearing problems in this case are often attributed to the middle ear disease, which resolves, and the child unfortunately is not referred for a hearing test.

Referral Criteria

It would be ideal if referrals could be based on a simple test in a pediatrician's office. Unfortunately, for children younger than 4 years such a test does not exist, except for an infant hearing screener based on the evoked response. As a result, many physicians observe a child's reaction to sound, such as a finger snap or kiss, in the office as an informal screening procedure. This practice is fraught with error because of the large variability of infants' responses to sound[3] and because of the excellent ability of hearing-impaired children to respond to minimal nonauditory cues during these types of tests. Pretesting with a bad test prevents patients from receiving an accurate test and delays diagnosis.

Parental concern should be foremost in referring a child for a hearing test. Parving[4] has shown that over one half of hearing losses in children are first noticed or suspected by parents. Risk factors such as family history of hearing loss, congenital perinatal infections, and abnormalities of the head[5] are also good reasons for referral, if one keeps in mind the fact that over one fourth of hearing-impaired children do not have any risk factors for hearing loss.[6] In addition, delays in speech and language development, however small, also indicate the need for testing. Children with repeated episodes of otitis media should be referred because of the high likelihood that residual serous fluid remains in the ears between episodes. This residual fluid can cause a conductive hearing loss that is just as handicapping as a sensorineural hearing loss. A failed screening test also warrants follow-up with a complete hearing evaluation. Finally, a hearing test is often a good initial evaluation when investigating academic or behavioral problems in school.

References
1. Starr A, Amlie RN, Martin WH, Sanders S: Development of auditory function in newborn infants revealed by auditory brainstem potentials. *Pediatrics* 1977;60:831.
2. Berrick JM, Thornton AR, Herrmann BS: ABR hearing screening of intensive care nursery graduates. *ASHA*(A) 1985;27:152.
3. Thompson G, Wilson W: Clinical application of visual reinforcement audiometry, in Mahoney T (ed): Early identification of hearing loss in infants. *Semin Hear* 1984;5:85.
4. Parving A: Hearing disabled children: Epidemiology and identification. *Scand Audiol* 1988;30:21.
5. American Academy of Pediatrics: Joint Committee on Infant Hearing position statement. *Pediatrics* 1982;80:496.
6. Stein L, Clark S, Kraus N: The hearing impaired infant: Patterns of identification and habilitation. *Ear Hear* 1983;4:232.

Neonatal Screening
Aaron Thornton, PhD

Points To Recall:
- *Speech and language development is critically dependent on hearing during the 1st year of life, so sensorineural hearing loss (SNHL) must be identified within the first 3 months.*
- *Pay attention to the mother and immediate family, as they are usually the first to identify SNHL, and never suggest that audiometric testing be deferred until the child is older.*
- *Risk factors can be used to identify infants who have the greatest likelihood for acquiring SNHL and should trigger testing by reliable audiometric procedures, such as auditory brain-stem response (ABR), within 3 months of the first suspicion.*
- *Audiometric screening of neonates by ABR instruments is reliable and accurate, and automated instruments make it possible to screen all newborns before discharge from the nursery.*

Considerations for Referral:
- *All neonates*
- *All infants presenting with risk factors, including caregiver concern*

The importance of hearing to the normal development of spoken language has been well defined for many decades, yet most educated people have only a vague understanding of the negative developmental effects of neonatal hearing loss. With an estimated incidence of deafness of only 1 in 1,500 live births, the average person has little opportunity to observe the slow language development of a deaf infant. Familiarity with deaf children is further limited, since they are often segregated into special educational classes. Likewise, we are isolated from direct knowledge of congenitally deafened adults, who prefer to associate with others in the deaf culture with whom they can communicate fluently in sign language. Consequently, parents of newly diagnosed infants often have no direct experience with deafness. Their most common experiences with childhood conductive hearing loss or lost hearing in adulthood are not comparable, and actually make it harder to understand the effects of neonatal hearing loss on speech and language development.

The critical foundations for spoken and written language are formed during the first 2 years of life. An infant who has been deprived of hearing will suffer significant delays in later development proportional to the severity of the hearing loss. Some will never achieve spoken language. For many of those identified early, within the first few weeks after birth, hearing aids and aural rehabilitation can dramatically change the course of development, sometimes making the difference between no spoken-language skills at the age of 2 years and normal speech and language acquisition. For the average deaf neonate, however, hearing aids will not be fitted, nor will habilitation and parental education begin until the child is 18 months of age—not because this has been determined to be the proper time, but because that is the average age at which severe to profound sensorineural hearing loss (SNHL) is diagnosed in developed countries.[1-3]

Because early manifestations of hearing loss are subtle, they are frequently dismissed as inattention, late development of speech, or slow mental development. The simple, intuitive tests are especially prone to error, most often serving to confirm the bias of the observer. Events that produce sounds also transmit vibrations and air movements, and they are usually accompanied by visible movements, shadows, and the reactions of nearby people. Therefore, when the alert infant responds, he or she is thought to have heard. The incessant activity of infants also increases the difficulty of determining the responsiveness to sound. The fact that hearing loss is seldom complete also helps to explain how the problem can be overlooked for such a long period. Unresponsiveness to softer sounds is easily rationalized, whereas a clear response to louder stimuli is likely to be taken as evidence of normal hearing. Responses to vibratory stimuli accompanied by softer sounds further reduce any suspicions of hearing loss, since sound awareness usually takes precedence over vibratory sensation for the hearing observer.

The mother and other close family members are the first to notice the symptoms of hearing loss,[1] but reassurances by well-meaning friends, relatives, and, too often, the family physician often delay the diagnosis by many months. In fact, perhaps as a misguided effort to mitigate the grief, there is a subsequent tendency to challenge the diagnosis of deafness, advising that the test might be wrong, that hearing tests cannot be accurately done in infancy, and that the parents should postpone testing until the child is older. For many parents, the inability of their child to speak at 2 or 3 years of age becomes increasingly difficult to ignore or rationalize, finally precipitating the request for a test. Multiply handicapped children are often delayed even longer, since their more apparent deficits seem to explain slow development.

Given the public's infrequent exposure to congenital deafness and the softness of symptoms during infancy, the cultural pattern of late identification of hearing loss is unlikely to improve so long as we depend on the parents and the family physician to refer infants for definitive testing. Screening is the obvious alternative, but that requires a consensus on the need and specific objectives; cooperation and coordination of community, state, and national resources; and, most important, a practical means of accomplishing the task. Until recently, one of the principal impediments to the testing of infants was the lack of a reliable and accurate procedure to assess hearing loss in the 1st year of life. The success of audiometric techniques widely available before the 1980s depended greatly on the skill of the examiner, and reliability was frequently established through serial testing, while the infant grew older and easier to assess. Once referred, the baby was evaluated repeatedly until the diagnosis was definitive, and the aggregate costs of the process, financial and emotional, could be significant.

In this context, a high-risk registry was devised to decrease the average age of diagnosis and control costs by reducing the size of the target population. In 1973, the Joint Committee on Infant Hearing Screening, consisting of representatives from the American Academy of Pediatrics, Academy of Otolaryngology—Head and Neck Surgery, American Nurses Association, and American Speech-Language-Hearing Association, identified five factors from the birth history that could be associated with significantly increased risk for hearing loss,[4] and they proposed registering any infant who met any one of the criteria at the time of birth and then following the child until a definitive diagnosis could be established through conventional testing.

The committee refined their position statement on the high-risk registry in 1982,[5] expanding the number of risk categories to seven. By 1987, variations on this theme had been tried on a statewide or regional basis in 12 states, and 7 other states were planning to try them.[6] On the surface, these developments were encouraging in that they indicated an increased awareness of infant hearing loss and public support for mass screening. On closer inspection, however, the registry concept has not lived up to its promise. More than 25% of all hearing-impaired infants do not manifest any of the risk factors proposed in the 1982 position statement,[5] which excludes them from the registry, decreases concerns, and perhaps delays identification.

Nevertheless, a program that identified upwards of 75% of the infants with handicapping SNHL would have been a major step forward, but, unfortunately, that figure represented an upper limit that could be achieved if a high-risk registry were fully implemented with 100% compliance. The actual performance has been dismal, largely due to the failure of parents of at-risk infants to take them for audiologic evaluation, despite multiple requests and the offer of free testing. The statistics are remarkably similar across programs. Approximately 10% of all neonates qualify for the high-risk register, but only about 10% of those (1% of the total) actually receive a hearing test as a result of the registry program. Consequently, we can estimate that only 7.5% of the neonates born with SNHL would be diagnosed at an earlier age as a result of high-risk-register screening programs.

The Joint Committee on Infant Hearing recently reaffirmed its faith in the high-risk register by issuing its 1990 position statement,[7] which expands the risk criteria from the 1982 statement and makes additional recommendations for the identification and management of hearing-impaired neonates and infants. As shown in **Appendix A**, the risk criteria are now considered separately for two age groups—neonates and infants—and there is now recognition of parental concern as a risk factor. The committee recommends completion of audiometric testing of at-risk neonates before discharge from the nursery and audiometric testing of at-risk infants within 3 months of identification. The purpose of early identification is to permit early habilitation, and the 1990 position statement stresses that early intervention services should be provided, in accordance with Public Law 99-457, which permits habilitative services to begin before all of the evaluation and assessment is completed. The roles of physician, audiologist, speech-language pathologist, and teacher of the hearing-impaired are outlined in the context of the individualized family service plan mandated by PL 99-457.

The 1990 position statement reflects the significant technologic advances in hearing testing that have been made since the 1973 and 1982 statements. For want of an accurate neonatal hearing test, the concept of a high-risk registry was originally developed to refer infants most likely to have SNHL into a serial-evaluation strategy at an earlier age. The 1990 position, however, clearly acknowledges that accurate audiometric testing can now be done before a neonate is discharged from the nursery, a capability that was nonexistent in 1973 and highly controversial in 1982. These same advances in testing methodology might also make the high-risk registry obsolete as a prescreening tool by making it possible to test every infant at birth.

The best-developed procedure for accurately testing the hearing of neonates and infants is the recording of the auditory brain-stem response (ABR). Initially, reliability and accuracy of ABR audiometry were critically dependent on the expertise of the examiner, who controlled a relatively complex instrument and visually interpreted a series of graphic results. As such, availability was limited and the cost for accurate results was too high for use in mass screening. As the technique has matured, however, adaptations have been made, with specific attention to decreasing the expertise needed to obtain accurate screening results.

Fully automated ABR neonatal hearing screeners that can operate unattended[8] can be used by indigenous nursery personnel to accurately screen hearing of neonates before discharge with very little incremental cost to the nursery. The cost per neonate tested over a 5-year period may be $2 to $3 for depreciation and maintenance of the instrument, $7 for disposables, and $10 to $15 for all other incremental overhead, including personnel. At $25 per neonate, identification of each case of SNHL would cost $37,500, assuming an incidence of 1/1,500. Each false-positive test result adds the cost of a follow-up test, and at an estimated rate of 2% and $500 per follow-up, another $15,000 can be added, bringing the total cost per identified SNHL up to $52,500. Nearly all of the neonates with SNHL from birth would be identified before leaving the nursery; but mass screening will be expected to miss as many as 13% of the infants with SNHL who acquire the hearing loss after leaving the nursery.[9]

Estimating the costs of a high-risk-registry program is more difficult, since the aggregate personnel costs are easily underestimated. The 10 high-risk criteria listed in **Appendix A** for neonates are relatively technical and complex, frequently requiring a judgment call from a professionally competent examiner. In practice, all of the relevant information must be gleaned from some combination of chart review, parental interview, and direct examination, easily totaling an incremental cost of $30 in hospital personnel per neonate ($45,000 for 1,500 neonates). At least 12% of these neonates can be expected to meet one or more of the expanded high-risk criteria and require a hearing screening, which could be as inexpensive as the one just described, costing $6300 per 1,500 neonates. Thus, the high-risk registry would cost $51,300, providing virtually no savings over the cost of testing every neonate, but it would miss as many as one of four of the neonates with SNHL, based on experience with the 1982 risk factors. Also, a program that screens at-risk neonates while still in the nursery will still miss the same 13% of infants who acquire hearing loss after discharge.

Space does not permit discussion of all the factors that might increase or decrease the specific costs of operating a risk registry or mass ABR screening, but it is clear that the simple expedient of testing every child should be considered when developing a program, as the amount of time and expertise needed to ascertain risk factors may actually be greater than that required to perform a definitive test. This is particularly true for the NICU, where the majority of neonates are at risk and the incidence of SNHL is as great as 2.5% for tertiary-care units.[10] Implementation of either alternative, mass screening or in-nursery screening of at-risk neonates, combined with aggressive follow-up, will ensure that neonates and infants will be diagnosed soon after birth so that hearing aids can be fitted and speech and language therapy can begin.

References
1. Parving A: Hearing disabled children: Epidemiology and identification. *Scand Audiol Suppl* 1988;30:21.
2. Stein L, Clark S, Kraus N: The hearing-impaired infant: Patterns of identification and habilitation. *Ear Hear* 1983;4:232.
3. Stein L, Jabaley T, Spitz R, et al: The hearing-impaired infant: Patterns of identification and habilitation revisited. *Ear Hear* 1990;11:201.
4. Joint Committee on Infant Hearing Screening: Supplementary statement. *ASHA* 1974;16:160.
5. Joint Committee on Infant Hearing: Position statement. *ASHA* 1982;24:1017.
6. Mahoney T: The ups and "downs" of high-risk hearing screening: The Utah statewide program, in Gerkin KP, Amochaev A (eds): *Semin Hear* 1987;8:155.
7. Joint Committee on Infant Hearing: Position statement. *AAO-HNS Bull* 1991;10:15.
8. Peters JG: An automated infant screener using advanced evoked response technology. *Hear J* 1986;39:25.
9. Davidson J, Hyde M, Ablerti P: Epidemiology of hearing impairment in childhood. *Scand Audiol Suppl* 1988;30:13.
10. Fria TJ: Identification of congenital hearing loss with the auditory brainstem response, in Jacobson J (ed): *The Auditory Brainstem Response*. San Diego: College-Hill Press, 1985, pp 317-334.

Discussion

Dr Hart: Five hundred thirty-two infants were tested for hearing loss by auditory brain-stem response (ABR) in the Phoenix Children's Hospital Intensive Care Nursery from 1989 through 1991. These infants met high-risk criteria similar to those recommended by the AAP/American Speech-Language-Hearing Association Committee on Hearing (**Appendix A**).

Overall, 32% of tested infants failed the ABR during these 3 years. Each year a higher percentage of eligible infants were actually tested, and with this there was an associated slight decrease, 24% failing during 1991. These percentages are higher than in some centers but are believed by some consultants to reflect the high incidence of very-high-risk infants in the population tested (eg, infants with birth weights < 1500 g represent 25% of admissions).

Although represented by smaller numbers, such risk factors as cytomegalovirus, hyperbilirubinemia, drugs of abuse, and congenital defects were associated with a failure rate of 54%. Finally, there was a relatively high incidence of unilateral mild hearing loss compared with bilateral and/or more severe loss.

Whether these findings will be permanent will be determined through follow-up testing at 3 to 6 months of age.

Dr Thornton: Over a 3-year period, we transported infants from the NICU to a sound-treated room. We found that the infants never make a mistake. If an infant has hearing, you can measure it. A baby who doesn't have an ABR (including cochlear potentials) doesn't have hearing. Examination error may explain many discrepancies across studies. For example, while visiting another nursery, I observed an experienced person testing. She was outstanding, but while we were standing there, the earphone slipped down on the infant's head to where it was no longer positioned across from the ear canal. So even with very good people, mistakes can easily go unnoticed. Well-designed instruments can greatly reduce the number of critical errors in testing.

Another problem is the noise in the nursery. We recommend taking infants to a sound-treated room or, alternatively, setting up the machine so that it will not test unless the background noise is within permissible limits.

We now have data on 800 NICU infants whom we followed in the last 5 years, in whom the total failure rate is about 6%. We found 2.5% have profound bilateral sensorineural hearing loss, the same as for other NICUs, and our false-positive rate is only 0.5%.

We test every infant who fails the screening within 24 hours in a sound-treated room and measure air- and bone-conduction thresholds on each ear for three frequencies. This lets us sort out permanent hearing loss, transient hearing loss, and measurement error. Two months later, it's too late.

I think the false-positive rate can actually be held under 1%, and even less than that in a well-baby nursery. As infants get older, the false-positive rate is likely to get higher, because they fuss around more and the machine is forced to test under marginal conditions. So the younger the infant, the better the test results we get.

The youngest infant we have tested was, I think, 28 weeks' gestational age. The ABR, if put into a series with others, is just as clear as for infants who are weeks older. I see no reason to wait for the child to get older.

Dr Yaffe: My question has to do with mathematics and the costs of neonatal screening. I am here as a public official, but also as an advocate for improved infant outcome. The Boston mathematics of $25 per infant multiplied by 4 million births in this country is not $50,000, but $100 million. How can neonatal screening be done for 4 million infants at $25 each?

Dr Klein: To identify how many children?

Dr Thornton: One in 1,500.

Dr Yaffe: The point is that you had better get this $25 cost down to the level of screening for phenylketonuria or the human immunodeficiency virus.

Dr Thornton: It would cost $52,000 to detect one severe hearing impairment. There are false-positive costs in there, too.

The $100 million is a lot of money, but not that much of the proportion that is spent on health care. However, $25 per birth is a fairly insignificant increase in obstetric costs.

Dr Hart: Dr Herrmann, you said that you believe the only valid test for newborns is the ABR. We concur. However, we have a problem with the 3-month follow-up, because frequently there has been a change in the doctor or the health care plan and the infant has been lost to follow-up.
Dr Herrmann: If an infant fails the hearing screening, it is important to have a complete evaluation before he or she leaves the nursery and to establish the cause of the failure.
Dr Brookhouser: There really are no good shortcuts for children aged 2 years and under. They need a thorough, well-done hearing test once you suspect something is going wrong. Stopping short of that results in inappropriate data.
Dr Klein: What do you recommend for the high-risk registry?
Dr Brookhouser: Universal testing of all NICU graduates with the ABR.
Dr Klein: Should those who fail be followed up?
Dr Brookhouser: Yes, with ABR follow-up.
Dr Klein: For now, the debate about screening all infants to pick up the 25% who have hearing loss will continue. But at the very least, there should be enforced testing of high-risk-registry infants and follow-up of those who fail.
Mr Gjerdingen: Dr Herrmann referred to deafness as the "invisible handicap," which people often do. I contend that it is not a handicap. It is a condition that causes a handicap. The handicap is what results if you don't do something about it. I do not consider Bonnie Tucker handicapped by deafness.

People define the categories of deafness and put profound deafness at the bottom, and then define profound deafness as a 90-dB hearing loss. But children with 90-dB hearing losses can learn to talk on the telephone, so we need some different categories before we can deal with children today.

Recognition of the Hearing-Impaired Patient in a Primary-Care Pediatric Practice

Jerome T. Combs, MD

Points To Recall:
- *All newborns can be screened for deafness.*
- *Language milestones can be monitored for all children.*
- *All patients can be screened for conductive hearing loss.*
- *Threshold audiometry is possible in a pediatrician's office.*

A primary-care provider has the first opportunity to recognize an infant or child with a hearing defect. The identification of such a patient should have high priority.

Twenty-five to 30 years ago, I was told several times during my training that it was not possible to test the hearing of newborn infants. I didn't question that statement. Fortunately, medical students and house staff are taught differently now. They know that certain infants—premies and those with sepsis, meningitis, hyperbilirubinemia, or other risk factors—should be screened for hearing defects. They are not taught to screen all newborns.

About 10 years ago, after attending a continuing medical education course that featured Dr Klein and Dr Charles Bluestone, I found myself reflecting on the problem of identifying deafness in newborns and recalled a childhood experience I would like to share. My father's avocation was raising hunting dogs, English setters. When I was 8 years old, I was watching my dad play with a litter of puppies. He spent hours checking their temperament, intelligence, and ability to smell. He did a doggie developmental exam, if you will, to select the pick of the litter, the pup most likely to become a field-trial champion. He knew that severe sensorineural (SN) hearing loss was inherited as an autosomal recessive trait in English setters and that if both pedigrees were free of deafness, some of the puppies still might be born deaf. The first thing he checked after they opened their eyes was their hearing. He picked up each pup in turn, cradled it in his palms, and made a kissing sound. Then he watched for the pup to grimace or blink its eyes as proof that it could hear. He explained that talking or whistling would not do, because the pup might be reacting to the expired air on its face.

All Newborns Can and Should Be Screened for Deafness

Downs[1] has documented that infants stimulated by sound will show a variety of behavioral responses, ranging from an eye blink to a Moro response with vigorous crying. In 1983, I used the kissing-sound technique to screen the infant daughter of Dr Frank Sansone, Chairman of the Department of Communication Disorders at Southern Connecticut State University. She rewarded us with a vigorous Moro response. He was delighted and went back to his laboratory to record the sonographic display on this sound, the acoustic kiss. He concluded that it is a rich sound and very appropriate for screening newborn infants.

Fig 1 compares the acoustic richness of this sound to a hand clap and a cheek click. The acoustic kiss has a broad frequency range and a harmonically distributed sound energy and is of ample duration to be an effective subjective screening test for newborn infants.

It takes about 10 seconds to screen a newborn for major bilateral hearing loss with this technique. This screening test is very appropriate to do, since severe SN hearing loss occurs in approximately 1 in 2,000 live births.[2] Additionally, this method of neonatal screening appears to be sensitive to moderate bilateral conductive hearing loss.

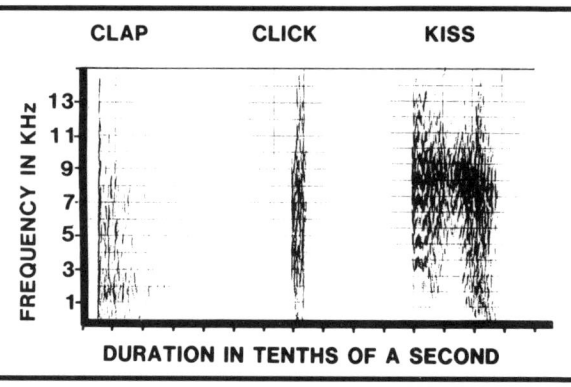

Fig 1. Sonographic display of three different sounds for subjective hearing screening of the newborn. Frequency by duration is shown, with the reflective intensity indicated by the darkness of the tracing.

I have an average-sized solo primary-care practice, and in the last 10 years five of my newborn patients have failed this test: an infant with severe bilateral SN hearing loss, one with cleft palate, and three who were subsequently proven to have otitis media by 2 months of age. Two of these infants needed ventilating tubes before 12 months of age.

Monitoring Language Milestones for All Infants and Toddlers

Screening for receptive and expressive language milestones during infancy and preschool years is also crucial in primary-care pediatrics. This has been made easier by the introduction of the Early Language Milestone (ELM) Scale, which has been documented to be of value[3] but is time-consuming and requires completion of an extensive form.

It seems to be more economical of time in a busy primary-care pediatric office to make ongoing observations during each of the well-baby visits recommended by the American Academy of Pediatrics. A simplified sequence of early auditory receptive and expressive milestones is shown in the Table. At-risk infants will be identified earlier with its use.

Table. Basic Early Auditory Responses.

Birth to 2 weeks:	Startles to auditory kiss
2 to 4 months:	Smiles to auditory kiss and coos
4 to 6 months:	Turns head to mother's voice
9 months:	Knows "No" and babbles
12 months:	Speaks first word (other than "Mama"/"Dada")
15 months:	Has two- or three-word vocabulary
18 months:	Speaks three to six words and points to ear/nose
24 months:	Speaks four dozen words and uses three-word sentences

This simplified approach will detect many infants and toddlers who need a more complete evaluation. They can then be evaluated with an ELM Scale and considered for referral to a speech and hearing center.

Screening All Patients for Conductive Hearing Loss

It is extremely important that all infants and children be screened for the conductive hearing loss associated with middle ear effusion (MEE). MEE in the first 2 or 3 years of life has a significant adverse effect on the cognitive and communicative abilities of children.[4] If a physician diagnoses acute otitis media (AOM) only in patients who present with earache, he or she is missing about half of the patients with AOM.[5] During the first 2 years of life, otalgia is apparent in only about 30% of infants with the disease.[5] The primary-care provider who never diagnoses MEE during well-baby examinations will miss about 25% of infants with this cause of conductive hearing loss.[6]

Tympanometry

Tympanometry is a useful technology for the primary-care provider, and every pediatrician should consider having a tympanometer in the office. One can measure the pressure behind the tympanic membrane (TM) with precision and accuracy. A normal tympanometry curve is about 95% predictive of a normal ear in a healthy child.[7] However, a recent large study reported that such curves occur in 15% of infants with AOM.[8] Additionally, it sometimes is impossible to perform tympanometry in a sick infant or toddler, because it is necessary to have a few moments of cooperation from the patient.

Studies of the ability of tympanometry to predict conductive hearing loss have been somewhat disappointing.[9] Yet much of what we have learned about otitis media in the last 30 years is the result of using this technology in clinical research[10]; tympanometry has served us well and will continue to do so in the future.

Acoustic Reflectometry

In 1984, a new technology for objective assessment of MEE was introduced by Teele and Teele.[11] The acoustic otoscope is a miniaturized sonar device that bounces sound energy of 80 dB off the TM and listens to the echo. The louder the echo, the more likely that MEE is present behind the TM.

Acoustic reflectometry is easier to perform than tympanometry. It requires no cooperation from the patient. The intensity of the reflected sound, the echo, is given in numerical units. Reflectivities of 0 to 3 are soft echos and generally predictive of no MEE. Echos of 4 and 5 are intermediate in value and may be normal or may be seen with a TM that is tense because of negative pressure caused by eustachian tube dysfunction. Intermediate reflectivities may also be found in ears that have a minimal amount of fluid. Reflectivities of 6 or more are predictive of MEE[12] unless the canal is impacted by wax.

Since the middle ear is a biophysical apparatus designed to conduct sound energy, it must obey the first and second laws of thermodynamics. Therefore, it follows that the louder the reflectivity, the more sound energy that bounces back off the TM; the less sound energy that gets through to the inner ear, the greater the conductive hearing loss.

Recently, Teele et al[13] proved that a reflectivity of 6 or more is predictive of a conductive hearing loss. Fig 2 is an idealized graphic representation of this relationship, adapted from these authors' data and modified by my experience with this technology. The exact shape of the curve depends on the frequency of the sound used for the test and the age of the patient.[14]

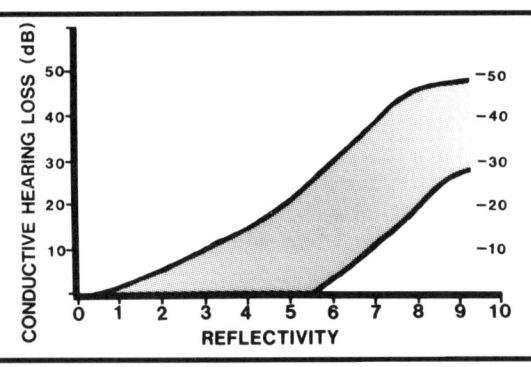

Fig 2. Probable correlation between acoustic reflectivity and conductive hearing loss. The curve is idealized from published data[13] and anecdotal experience.

I find the acoustic otoscope extraordinarily helpful in the objective management of MEE in infants and children. During the last 7 years, I have screened for conductive hearing loss in every patient I have seen in my office by using the acoustic otoscope.

It should be noted that, whereas acoustic reflectometry with a recorder is capable of excellent precision,[15] this technology is very sensitive to user technique.[16] Falsely low reflectivities are very likely if it is used in a casual manner.

Office-Based Audiometry

For years I puzzled over the problems of doing reliable audiometry in a busy primary-care pediatric office. I felt that I needed a good technician, an accurate instrument, and a soundproof room; the room seemed to be the most difficult to acquire. About 2 years ago, it dawned on me that my office is a quiet room when I'm not in it and that the mother of a hearing-impaired child would be a good person to train as a technician. Now I have an excellent technician who does threshold audiometry two afternoons a week when I am not in the office. This has worked out very well, and we get very satisfactory results.

I believe that virtually every practice has a dedicated mother of a hearing-impaired child. If not, a letter to the Alexander Graham Bell Association for the Deaf [see **Appendix B**] would help locate the nearest chapter of the society and a parent who would be interested in being trained to do reliable threshold audiometry independently on a part-time basis.

Case Presentation

J.T., a 7½-year-old boy, was seen for a physical examination because the school psychologist had diagnosed attention-deficit disorder and believed the boy should receive medication. J.T. had no history of earache, but had just gotten over a "cold" that had lasted 3 or 4 weeks. His left TM looked normal and the right was opaque. The diagnosis of unilateral otitis media with effusion would easily have been missed by a physician who did not do pneumatic otoscopy routinely or did not have tympanometry or acoustic reflectometry equipment at hand. At his first visit, J.T. had a mild unilateral hearing loss. He was put on amoxicillin, 250 mg tid, and given a note for school. When he returned 4 weeks later, he had normal ears and normal hearing. In the interim, he had stopped acting-out in school, and he continues to do well academically. Obviously, the school psychologist had failed to take the boy's past behavioral history into consideration and had made an incorrect diagnosis.

This case demonstrates how disabling even a modest, transient, unilateral, conductive hearing loss can be. Bess[17] has pointed out that the unilaterally hearing-impaired child will either exhibit withdrawn behavior or act-out in the classroom, and a recent study[18] has suggested that middle ear disease in school-age children can result in hyperactivity that mimics attention-deficit disorder.

It should be apparent how helpful it is to have tympanometry, acoustic reflectometry, and threshold audiometry in primary-care pediatric offices.

References

1. Downs MP: Testing hearing in infancy and early childhood, in Freeman M, Ward PH (eds): *Deafness in Childhood*. Nashville: Vanderbilt University Press, 1967, pp 25-33.
2. Proctor CA, Proctor B: Understanding hereditary nerve deafness. *Arch Otolaryngol* 1967;85:23.
3. Coplan J, Gleason JR: Quantifying language development from birth to 3 years using the Early Language Milestone Scale. *Pediatrics* 1990;86:963.
4. Teele DW, Klein JO, Chase C, et al: Otitis media in infancy and intellectual ability, school achievement, speech, and language at 7 years. *J Infect Dis* 1990;162:685.
5. Arola M, Ruuskanen O, Ziegler T, et al: Clinical role of respiratory virus infection in acute otitis media. *Pediatrics* 1990;86:848.
6. Marchant CD, Shurin PA, Tutihasi MA, et al: Detection of asymptomatic otitis media in early infancy, in Lim DJ (ed): *Recent Advances in Otitis Media*. Philadelphia: Decker, 1984, pp 32-33.
7. Bluestone CD, Klein JO: *Otitis Media in Infants and Children*. Philadelphia: WB Saunders Co, 1988, p 85.

8. Pichichero M, Aronovitz GH, Gooch WM, et al: Comparison of cefuroximine axetil, cefaclor, and amoxicillin-clavulanate potassium suspensions in acute otitis media in infants and children. *South Med J* 1990;83:1174.
9. Bess F: Audiometric approaches used in the identification of middle ear disease in children, in Kavanagh JF (ed): *Otitis Media and Child Development*. Parkton, Md: York Press, 1986, pp 73-77.
10. Bluestone CD, Klein JO: *Otitis Media in Infants and Children*. Philadelphia: WB Saunders Co, 1988, pp 82-92.
11. Teele DW, Teele J: Detection of middle ear effusion by acoustic reflectometry. *J Pediatr* 1984;104:832.
12. Lampe RM, Schwartz RH: Diagnostic value of acoustic reflectometry in children with acute otitis media. *Pediatr Infect Dis J* 1989;8:59.
13. Teele DW, Stewart IA, Teele JH, et al: Acoustic reflectometry for assessment of hearing loss in children with middle ear effusion. *Pediatr Infect Dis J* 1990;9:870.
14. Combs JT: Change of acoustic reflectivity with age. *J Pediatr* 1990;117:80.
15. Combs JT: Precision of acoustic reflectometry with recorder in acute otitis media. *Pediatr Infect Dis J* 1988;7:329.
16. Combs JT: Predictive value of the angle of acoustic reflectivity tracings. *Pediatr Infect Dis J* 1991;10:212.
17. Bess FH: The unilaterally hearing-impaired child: A final comment. *Ear Hear* 1986;7:52.
18. Adesman AR, Altshuler LA, Lipkin PH, et al: Otitis media in children with learning disabilities and in children with attention deficit disorder with hyperactivity. *Pediatrics* 1990;85:442.

Screening School-Age Children for Auditory Function

Fred H. Bess, PhD

Points To Recall:
- *The prevalence of hearing loss and middle ear disease among schoolchildren is high.*
- *The availability, comprehensiveness, and quality of school screening programs vary dramatically from school to school.*

Consideration for Referral:
- *Failure of screening for hearing loss and/or middle ear disease*

Identification audiometry is an important component of any comprehensive management strategy for hearing-impaired children. It is a technique designed to separate in a simple, rapid, and inexpensive manner those children who have an auditory disorder from those who do not. Identification audiometry is a preventive measure that emphasizes early detection and prompt intervention and/or habilitation. In children, the objective is to eliminate or minimize any hearing loss that could affect learning as soon as an impairment is detected. Screening is not a diagnostic procedure and does not offer information relative to the degree, the type, or the cause of the impairment. It is merely the first step in a much more comprehensive hearing-conservation program that includes a minimum of aspects such as medical, audiologic, and educational services.

When screening for school-age children is being considered, it is first important to recognize that hearing tests do not inform us about the adequacy of the middle ear, nor does immittance give us information about hearing level. The ineffectiveness of pure-tone audiometry for detecting middle ear disease was demonstrated in several studies.[1,2] If the goal is to identify hearing loss, pure-tone audiometry should be the test of choice; however, if the goal is to detect middle ear disease, electroacoustic immittance should be the screening tool.

Prevalence of Hearing Loss and Middle Ear Disease

Hearing loss resulting from either middle ear or sensorineural pathology affects a large number of school-age children in the United States. It is estimated that there are about 44,000 schoolchildren with severe to profound hearing losses and another 950,000 children with losses in the mild to moderate categories.[3] The well-known Pittsburgh study[4] has reported that about 50 of every 1,000 schoolchildren (5%) exhibit reduced hearing levels in either one or both ears. Silverman and Lane[5] have estimated that 2.5 million schoolchildren exhibit some degree of hearing loss. The prevalence of middle ear disease is discussed by Dr Klein in this publication.

Status of School Screening Programs

The practice of school screening has existed for more than 60 years, and every state in the nation conducts some form of hearing screening in schools, but fewer than half of the states have passed legislation requiring such screening. The lack of uniformity among state screening programs is demonstrated by different agencies responsible for screening, variations in criteria for children to be tested, differences in screening techniques, and varying qualifications of personnel who conduct the screening programs. About one half of the states incorporate some type of immittance measure into their screening procedure.

Who Is Responsible?

Ideally, the state department of education should coordinate the periodic screening of all schoolchildren and provide for the necessary educational, audiologic, and rehabilitative follow-up. The state department of health should coordinate the activities of identification audiometry, threshold measurement, and medical follow-up for those students who fail the screening tests.

Personnel

Volunteers, nurses, audiologists, speech-language pathologists, graduate students in speech and hearing, and even secretaries have been designated to conduct the testing. To ensure quality programs, only professionals trained in audiology should coordinate and supervise hearing-conservation programs. Volunteers and lay groups can be used in a supportive manner such as to promote the screening programs. Audiologists should administer the screening programs and trained audiometrists or technicians should perform the actual screening.

Who Should Be Screened?

It is not economically feasible to mass-screen all children in the schools; therefore, a decision must be made to identify the target population. Most programs have concentrated their annual screening efforts on children of nursery-school age through grade 3. In fact, screening in these grades is recommended in the guidelines of the American Speech-Language-Hearing Association (ASHA).[6] Following grade 3, children may be screened at 3- to 4-year intervals. ASHA recommends that children at risk for hearing loss be screened annually. This includes children who 1) repeat a grade, 2) require special education programs, 3) are new to the school system, 4) were absent during a previously scheduled screening examination, 5) failed a threshold test during the previous year, 6) have speech or language problems or obvious difficulty in communication, 7) are suspected of having hearing impairment or a medical problem associated with hearing impairment, and 8) are at risk for noise exposure.

Equipment, Calibration, and the Test Environment

An important component of any identification program is the audiometric equipment used in the screening. The equipment for pure-tone screening should be simple, sturdy, and portable. Care must be taken to ensure that the equipment performs satisfactorily and is calibrated periodically. Screening must also be conducted in a quiet environment, preferably with carpet and curtains and free from external noise from playgrounds, heavy traffic, or railroad tracks.

Identification Tests and Procedures

The individual pure-tone screening test is the most effective approach to screening hearing. In 1961, a comprehensive monograph developed by the National Conference on Identification Audiometry (NCIA)[7] outlined general guidelines for individual pure-tone screening. These guidelines recommended that the test frequencies in screening consist of 500, 1000, 2000, 4000, and 6000 Hz and that the screening occur in a sound-treated environment. More recently, ASHA developed a set of guidelines[6] in recognition that sound-treated rooms are not possible in most schools. The ASHA guidelines specify that a manual audiometer be used; that the test frequencies include 1000, 2000, and 4000 Hz, and that 500 Hz be used if acoustic immittance is not part of the screening protocol; and that the screening level for all frequencies be 20 dB hearing level. Lack of response to the recommended screening levels at any frequency in either ear represents a failure. All children who fail should be rescreened, preferably within the same test session but never later than 2 weeks afterward. Those who fail the rescreening should be referred to an audiologist for comprehensive evaluation.

According to Wilson and Walton,[8] this technique is 95% accurate. In their study of 8,000 schoolchildren, 77.9% of the group passed the initial screen. The 11.3% of the children who failed the initial screen but passed the rescreen illustrate the importance of retesting those who fail; 10.8% of the children failed both the initial screen and the rescreen.[8] According to Roeser and Northern,[9] the respective sensitivity and specificity for these data were 63% and 97%. Hence, 97% of the normal-hearing children were identified correctly; however, only 63% of the children with hearing loss were correctly identified, leaving 37% improperly classified as not having hearing loss.

Identification of Middle Ear Disease in Schoolchildren

There has long been interest in the use of electroacoustic immittance measures to identify middle ear disease in children. Even though specific guidelines for immittance screening were unavailable until recently, this technique has gained widespread popularity as a screening instrument. Several factors have contributed to the interest in immittance as a screening tool, including the ease and rapidity with which it can obtain accurate information, the high prevalence of middle ear disease, the relative ineffectiveness of pure-tone audiometry to detect a middle ear problem, and the growing concern for possible psychoeducational complication associated with middle ear disease.[10]

In 1977, a special task force studied the use of immittance measures in screening for middle ear disease.[11] The task force recognized the potential value of immittance screening but concluded after reviewing the available data that mass screening with immittance was not recommended. The task force did, however, recommend screening of high-risk populations such as Native Americans, those with sensorineural hearing loss, developmentally delayed or mentally retarded children, and children with Down syndrome, cleft palate, or other craniofacial anomalies.

A problem with immittance screening has been establishing appropriate pass/fail criteria. The pass/fail criteria of ASHA and the special task force have resulted in unacceptably high referral rates (32% to 36%).

Development of New Screening Guidelines for Hearing Loss and Middle Ear Disease

Recently, ASHA developed new guidelines for screening children that include a measure for both hearing loss and middle ear disease.[1,2] The screening protocol involves the use of case history, visual inspection of the ear canal and drum, identification audiometry, and tympanometry. For history, the protocol simply considers recent evidence of otalgia or otorrhea. Visual inspection via otoscopy is performed to identify gross abnormalities. For identification audiometry, ASHA recommends using the protocol described earlier.[6] For tympanometry, the recommendations for referral are 1) flat tympanogram and equivalent ear-canal volume outside normal range; 2) low static admittance on two successive occurrences in a 4- to 6-week interval; and 3) abnormally wide tympanometric width on two successive occurrences in a 4- to 6-week interval. Failure of the screen should result in an audiologic evaluation and a medical consultation. Because these guidelines are so new, data pertaining to the performance of the protocol are limited.

Roush and co-workers[13] examined only the tympanometry component of the revised ASHA guidelines in a large population of 3- and 4-year-old children. The "gold standard" was pneumatic otoscopy by a validated otoscopist. The resulting sensitivity and specificity were very good. The positive predictive value, on the other hand, was only 69%, meaning that only about two thirds of the children who failed the screen were classified otologically as abnormal. These data suggest that although the immittance component appears to have potential for detecting middle ear disease, more research is needed before we can draw any definitive conclusions about these guidelines.

References

1. Eagles EL, Wishik SM, Doerfler LG, et al: Hearing sensitivity and related factors in children. *Laryngoscope* 1963;suppl:1-220.
2. Melnick W, Eagles EL, Levine HS: Evaluation of a recommended program of identification audiometry with school-age children. *J Speech Hear Disord* 1964;29:3.
3. Lenich JK, Bernstein ME, Nevitt A: Educational audiology: A proposal for training and accreditation. *Lang Speech Hear Serv Schools* 1987;18:344.
4. Eagles EL, Wishik SM, Doerfler LG: Hearing sensitivity and ear disease in children: A prospective study. *Laryngoscope* 1967;suppl:1-274.
5. Silverman SR, Lane HS: Deaf children, in Davis H, Silverman SR (eds): *Hearing and Deafness*, ed 3. New York: Holt Rinehart Winston, 1970, pp 384-425.
6. American Speech-Language-Hearing Association: Guidelines for identification audiometry. *ASHA* 1985;27:49.
7. Darley FL (ed): Identification audiometry. *J Speech Hear Disord* 1961;suppl 9:26.
8. Wilson WR, Walton WK: Identification audiometry accuracy: Evaluation of a recommended program for school-age children. *Lang Speech Hear Serv Schools* 1974;5:8.
9. Roeser RJ, Northern JL: Screening for hearing loss and middle ear disorders, in Roeser RJ, Downs MD (eds): *Auditory Disorders in School Children*, ed 2. New York: Thieme Medical Publishers, 1988, pp 72-77.
10. Bess FH, Humes LE: *Audiology: The Fundamentals*. Baltimore: Williams & Wilkins Co, 1990, pp 173-175.

11. Harford ER, Bess FH, Bluestone CD, Klein JO: *Impedance Screening for Middle Ear Disease in Children.* New York: Grune & Stratton, 1977, pp 3-8.
12. American Speech-Language-Hearing Association: Guidelines for screening for hearing impairments and middle ear disorders. *ASHA* 1990;32:17.
13. Roush J, Drake A, Sexton JV: Identification of middle ear disease in young children: A comparison of tympanometric screening protocols. *Ear Hear*, in press.

Discussion

Dr Thornton: Dr Combs, you mentioned training an office technician to do the testing. Who trains the technician? Who trains the trainer? Even with well-trained and highly supervised, licensed people, many mistakes can be made. I would not want to recommend that a pediatrician train a hearing-impaired person to conduct the tests.

Dr Combs: The parent of a hearing-impaired child who has a vested interest in this matter has been doing screening audiometry on a volunteer basis for one of our local organizations for years and is an active member of the Alexander Graham Bell Association. I sent her to a 1-day training program. She does threshold testing.

Dr Thornton: My recommendation, in any state where audiology is licensed, is that screening should be done by licensed audiologists. They can be hired on a part-time basis; referral can be set up with a local hospital. I don't think we should ignore the fact that we have probably the best audiologic services of any country in the world.

Dr Klein: Are you denying the validity of office screening?

Dr Thornton: Yes, unless it is 100% supervised by a physician.

Dr Bess: Sometimes, in an office setting, you can look at the secondary manifestations of hearing loss, such as speech/language development, and I believe Dr Combs mentioned the use of the Early Language Milestone (ELM) Scale or something similar. That is a viable alternative for primary-care providers. I recommend it, and I also recommend referring the patient for an audiologic evaluation. The ELM is not a direct test of hearing, but it is better than nothing at all.

Dr Ruben: I think we are getting down to the fundamental dilemma of American medicine. Yes, we built the best machine around, but who can get to it? I agree with Dr Thornton and Dr Bess. However, I think Dr Combs has a substantive issue.

Many children in this country do not have access to a Dr Combs or a Dr Thornton. They do not have access to a pediatric otolaryngologist. They are unable to get a screening test, let alone a definitive audiogram. The children of the City of New York do not have sufficient audiologists within the municipal hospital system to test them. There are long waiting lists and the end result is that the children are not tested.

It should be noted that in a society where there is access, what Drs Thornton and Bess state is fine. I am concerned that children in the inner city or on the reservation do not have access.

Ms Tucker: You should be aware that there may be licensure requirements in some states for people who are going to do any type of hearing screening. If a physician is not supervising, the person must have some kind of credentials to do this.

Dr Stool: The basic tool that the physician uses is still otoscopy, and this is his or her primary means of contact with the patient. Some are recommending that the primary-care physician obtain a pneumatic diagnostic otoscope with either a wall connection or a rechargeable battery and a halogen light, that this is the minimum requirement for screening in children. But it is the educated eye that is most important, along with the history, the physical examination, and the laboratory work. The laboratory work of impedance measurements provides a backup for the eye. In other words, if the impedance is off, you go back and look again. And in most instances, the child who has a fairly asymptomatic middle ear effusion will be identified.

Dr Brookhouser: I applaud Dr Combs's belief that a primary-care physician should be concerned about the hearing of anyone who comes to his or her office. The important distinction is between screening and definitive audiometry in the office. We should restrict the performance of a nonlicensed individual to simple screening tests. If children fail the screening, they should be referred for more definitive evaluation.

One also ought to screen with history. Every time the parents bring the child in, they should be asked about the milestone developments in the child's auditory awareness.

Dr Thornton: Pediatricians should support school screening programs, because they depend on them tremendously for referrals. Parents sometimes question whether they should follow up a failed screening at school, and it is important to bolster the school program by taking the time to talk to the school personnel and becoming familiar with the screening program.

Dr Stool: Physicians should understand the test that is being performed in their community. As Dr Bess says, every community has different criteria, and if you are going to see patients, you should learn the school criteria for pass/fail, and it should be made very clear to the family that this is not an intelligence test.

Perhaps another term could be used instead of "failing the school screening test"; the proper terminology for the school to use is "identifying the child with a potential problem," not "pass/fail." Parents associate failing with "dumbness," and these are not "dumb" children.

Dr Ruben: Several years ago, the European Economic Community brought together a group of people to address the failures in screening programs worldwide. Our consensus was that a single technique would not work, but that a number of different strategies should be simultaneously enacted, including high-risk registries, the testing of outcomes, routine testing of very-high-risk infants, public education, and continuing education of primary physicians and parents [Ruben, *Acta Otolaryngol Suppl* 1991;482:127].

Dr Thornton: I would say the most important message is to support any community hospital or group in developing a screening program of whatever type it is able to put together. Second, where there is suspicion of hearing loss, have the hearing tested. There is no reason to have a parent or a child wait for a hearing test.

Session IV—
Effects of Hearing Loss on Development

Speech and Language Development
Lynne V. Feagans, PhD

Point To Recall:
- *Physicians must be sensitive to possible hearing and speech impairment, even in children not in "risk" categories.*

Considerations for Referral:
- *Frequent or prolonged otitis media*
- *Speech delay*

The most consistent and persistent effects of hearing loss in infancy and early childhood are the effects on speech and language development. To describe these effects briefly, I will review four topics: 1) two types of hearing loss, with a focus on conductive hearing loss; 2) risk factors associated with hearing loss; 3) possible short- and long-term effects on speech and language development as related to the kind and duration of hearing loss; and finally 4) the physician's role in identification and referral for diagnosis and treatment of children with possible speech and language delay due to hearing loss.

Two Types of Hearing Loss

Two major types of hearing loss are associated with speech and language problems in infancy and early childhood. The first is sensorineural hearing loss, which is related to actual structural abnormalities or damage to the inner ear structures themselves, generally resulting in a permanent hearing loss often called "nerve deafness." Most children with this kind of loss are born with it, although it is estimated that 20% to 30% of affected children acquire the hearing loss after birth.[1] It is estimated that 3.5 per 1,000 infants in a well-baby nursery have a sensorineural hearing loss.[1] It also has been shown that the guidelines established by the Joint Committee on Infant Hearing (1982)[2] will identify only about half the infants with such a hearing loss. The others have no known risk factors that would place them at risk for hearing loss and subsequent language and speech problems.[3]

Another large group of children have conductive hearing loss due to fluid in the middle ear. These are children with otitis media, which is almost always accompanied by some mild to moderate hearing loss due to the middle ear fluid. This fluid may last several days or months and is often recurrent during the period that children are acquiring speech and language skills. Estimates range widely as to the incidence of otitis media in young children, but most studies suggest that at least 75% of children have at least one episode in the preschool years and that as many as one third of young children have at least three episodes a year.[4] Although a conductive hearing loss does not usually lead to permanent hearing loss, it is of concern to speech and language professionals because there is a high incidence of otitis media and because the hearing loss associated with it occurs most frequently during such a critical period of speech and language development.

Risk Factors for Poor Speech and Language Development Due to Hearing Loss

Any mild, moderate, or severe hearing loss in infancy and early childhood can have a severe effect on the development of speech and language.[5] Although there is great variability among individuals in the exact nature of these effects, the greater the hearing loss within the speech frequencies, the more overall delay in speech and language development. Early diagnosis and immediate treatment of the hearing loss are the best ways to prevent severe developmental delays in speech and language.

Although there are risk factors that physicians can routinely consider, these factors can only identify up to three fourths of the infants with a hearing loss. The Joint Commission on Infant Hearing guidelines for health care providers list the risk factors for sensorineural hearing loss (**Appendix A**).

Hearing loss in the other one fourth of children will be first noticed by parents and will require a clinically sensitive physician to detect the early, subtle risk factors, especially with mild to moderate loss.

Although Dr Klein[6] elaborates on the risk factors associated with a conductive hearing loss, there is one risk factor that will be elaborated here because the children are increasing in numbers rapidly: attendance at day care. More than half the women in this country who have a child under the age of 2 years are working full time. This percentage has doubled in less than 15 years, and it has become increasingly important to examine the health of infants and children in day care.

The Figure shows the proportion of illness for the children in the Penn State Health and Daycare Study.[7] Fifty-eight infants and toddlers have been examined independently by a nurse and physician each week for several years. Although there is large seasonal variation, the children have otitis media about 20% to 30% of the time. This is certainly more than in other studies, although it may be due to greater illness in day care or to greater documentation of disease. Most other studies of otitis media have examined the children once every other month or even less frequently. Most of the otitis media documented here is silent; that is, the children exhibit few if any symptoms of disease or hearing loss.

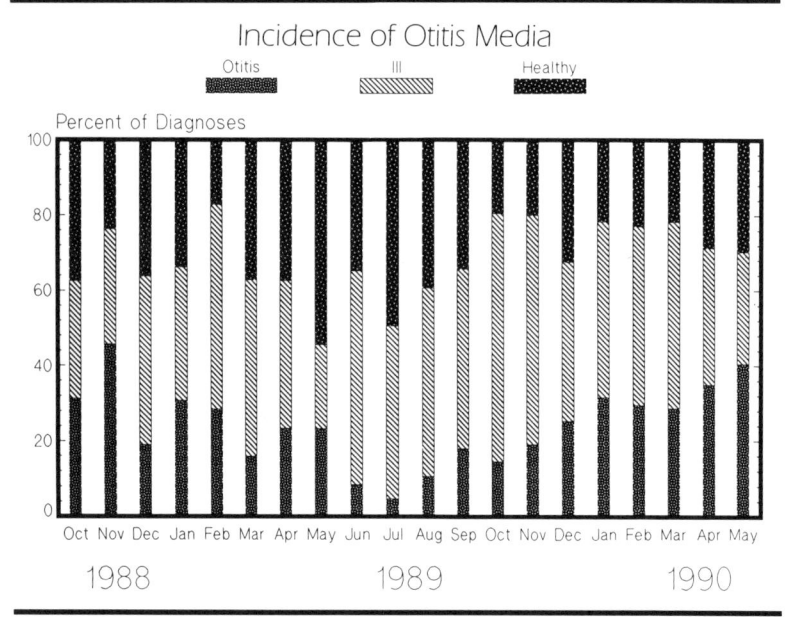

Figure. Incidence of otitis media and other illness in 58 children attending day care in central Pennsylvania, 1988-1990.

Hearing Loss and Speech and Language Development (Especially Conductive Hearing Loss)

The effects of sensorineural hearing loss early in life are well documented. There can be mild to profound delays in the acquisition of speech and language.[5] The effects of the mild to moderate intermittent hearing loss due to otitis media on speech and language are still argued among professionals. The hearing loss during otitis media is usually between 20 dB and 30 dB, although greater loss occasionally occurs.[8] Putting one's fingers into one's ears reveals the kind of loss these children experience. In a quiet environment with optimal input, such a loss should not affect speech discrimination. But in a noisy environment or one in which language is not clearly spoken, it can have an effect, even on an adult. Young children who experience this kind of loss may be at even greater risk because they are acquiring the rudiments of the oral-language system.

Length and Severity of Hearing Loss

Although many studies have found a relationship between otitis media and hearing loss and other studies have found a relationship between otitis media and language skills, there is still very little information about the frequency and severity of otitis media young children must have in order to place them at risk for developmental problems. Most of the best research studies use one of two criteria in classifying children at risk. First, some studies examine the number of episodes of otitis per year. The commonly accepted number that places a child in the high-otitis or at-risk group is three or more episodes per year. Because episodes can be very short or very long, especially with respect to the duration of effusion in the middle ear, the other common measure is the duration of effusion per year. Many physicians use as a rule of thumb 2.5 to 3 months, after which time they refer the child to an ENT specialist or for hearing and speech evaluation. Yet all these measures are somewhat intuitive and not based on the best scientific evidence. At present, they are the best rough guides to potential problems in speech and language.

The following aspects of language and speech have been purported to be affected by an intermittent hearing loss in early childhood, but can also be associated with a sensorineural hearing loss.

Expressive Language

Most studies of the short- and long-term effects of otitis media have examined expressive language problems. Although many of the studies were retrospective in nature and thus suspect with regard to experimental rigor, several prospective studies have now documented both short- and long-term expressive language problems in children as young as 2 years of age.[9-11] These problems can be divided into three major categories: syntactic, semantic, and pragmatic.

Syntactic problems are those of grammatical structures and morphology of the language. Some studies have found that otitis-prone children use less sophisticated sentences and even ungrammatical or incomplete sentences. Although all children use some ungrammatical sentences, otitis-prone children may use more of them and for a longer period. Semantic problems relate to the meaning elements in the language. Studies have found that otitis-prone children have a delayed acquisition of words and may have a smaller vocabulary than other children. Pragmatics is the use of language in context, at the discourse level; conversing and telling a narrative or story are examples. Children with a history of otitis media have been found to have more trouble telling a story they have previously comprehended than do non-otitis-prone children in kindergarten and second grade, many years after their hearing has returned to normal.[9] Pragmatic skills are particularly important when children enter school, because teachers expect them to be able to engage in conversational dialogue and to tell stories and recount events.

Receptive Language Problems

Less research is available on the receptive language problems of otitis-prone children, mainly because these are less obvious and harder to assess. A young child's understanding of language can be very difficult to assess. Most studies report a language score that may include mostly expressive language but also some receptive skills. These receptive problems can also be divided into syntactic, semantic, and pragmatic comprehension skills. Menyuk[12] has reported poorer syntactic comprehension and poorer receptive vocabulary (semantic) scores in high- versus low-otitis children. These poorer skills have been found even after the incidence of otitis media is diminished in the later preschool and early elementary-school period. The only study to examine pragmatic comprehension skills[9] found no effects on comprehension of narrative stories in school-age children who had had high otitis media in infancy and early childhood. This study did find that children who had had otitis media in early childhood paid less attention to their teachers in the classroom and to other academic activities, indicating that otitis-prone children may not attend to or listen to language as well as non-otitis-prone children.

Speech Problems

Speech problems have been documented in a few studies of otitis media. These generally fall under the rubric of poor phonology or articulation. It is still not clear what aspects of speech are most affected, and studies report some differing results.[13] In general, otitis-prone children are thought to be less intelligible as young children, and the higher-frequency sounds such as *sh* and *f* might be more affected.

Identification and Referral

Despite the existence of guidelines for identifying hearing loss and risk of chronic otitis media, more than half of the children with hearing loss cannot be identified through such guidelines. Thus, physicians need to be sensitive to the signs of speech and language problems to identify children at risk for hearing loss. It is difficult to identify most children with a mild to moderate hearing loss at an early age. They may exhibit normal developmental milestones until about the age of 2 years, when language fails to keep pace. Some of the following proposed guidelines for screening by physicians include factors that are associated not only with hearing loss but also with other general delays in speech and language.

One year of age. At 1 year of age, children generally can comprehend some words and are particularly attentive to speech. If parents report that their child does not respond to sounds or speech or responds only when the signal is very loud, referral should be made, especially if the physician can verify this lack of responsiveness on a well-baby visit. When the child is between 1 and 2 years of age, parents may report that the child tries to turn up the sound on the TV. This is another clue that some hearing loss may be present.

Two years of age. At 2 years of age, a child should be able to speak in words that parents can identify, even if they are unintelligible to a stranger. Children who have only a few words and do not appear to comprehend simple commands and words such as *no* should be referred for further evaluation. Children who have an uncharacteristic voice pattern could have a hearing loss in the high speech frequencies. Such children often speak in a low, unmodulated voice because they do not hear the high sounds of speech. Parent report of such a strange voice, accompanied by poor or unintelligible speech, also warrants referral.

Three years of age. Three-year-olds should be speaking in short phrases and be able to converse well and intelligibly. A child who is still speaking only in two-word phrases should be referred. Children who are still largely unintelligible, especially if this is verified by physician and parent, should also be referred for evaluation. Often a mild hearing loss (20-30 dB) can be undetected in infants and toddlers because hearing tests at these early ages can be difficult as well as unreliable. This kind of loss is still significant. Thus, even if results of a previous hearing test were within normal limits, another test should be given at age 3 years, when audiologic procedures are more successful and reliable.

Additional Guidelines for Referral for Conductive Hearing Loss

Prolonged conductive hearing loss at any age younger than 3 years may have significant effects on speech and language. Although there is still controversy about which children experience the hearing loss and for how long, some informal guidelines have been established for referral for an audiologic evaluation. Children who have had at least three documented episodes of otitis media in 1 year should have a hearing evaluation, preferably during the current episode. Because so many episodes are undetected, children who are known to have had three in a year may actually have had many more. Children who have had an episode of otitis media that lasts longer than 6 weeks should also have a hearing test. This is especially important with bilateral otitis media.

References

1. Matkin ND: Re-evaluating our approach to evaluation: Demographics are changing—Are we?, in Bess FH (ed): *Hearing Impairment in Children.* Parkton, Md: York Press, 1988, pp 101-111.
2. Joint Committee on Infant Hearing: Position statement. *ASHA* 1982;24:1017.
3. Glossack ME, McKennan KX, Levine SC: Differential diagnosis of sensorineural hearing loss in children, in Bess FH (ed): *Hearing Impairment in Children.* Parkton, Md: York Press, 1988, pp 1-14.
4. Feagans L, Blood I, Tubman JG: Otitis media: Models of effects and implications for intervention, in Bess FH (ed): *Hearing Impairment in Children.* Parkton, Md: York Press, 1988, pp 347-374.
5. Matkin ND: The role of hearing in language development, in Kavanagh JF (ed): *Otitis Media and Child Development.* Parkton, Md: York Press, 1986, pp 3-11.
6. Klein JO: Risk factors for otitis media in children, in Kavanagh JF (ed): *Otitis Media and Child Development.* Parkton, Md: York Press, 1986, pp 45-51.
7. Feagans LV, Blood I: Attention to language in day care attending children: A mediating factor in the developmental effects of otitis media. Presented at First International Congress of Behavioral Medicine, Uppsala, Sweden, June 1990.

8. Bess FH, McConnell FE: *Audiology, Education and the Hearing-Impaired Child.* St Louis: CV Mosby Co, 1981.
9. Feagans L, Sanyal M, Henderson F, et al: Middle ear disease in early childhood and later language skills. *J Pediatr Psychol* 1987;12:581.
10. Teele DW, Klein JO, Rosner BA: Otitis media with effusion during the first three years of life and development of speech and language. *Pediatrics* 1984;74:282.
11. Friel-Patti S, Finitzo-Heber T, Conti G, Brown CK: Language delay in infants associated with middle ear disease and mild, fluctuating hearing impairment. *Pediatr Infect Dis* 1982;1:104.
12. Menyuk P: Predicting speech and language problems with persistent otitis media, in Kavanagh JF (ed): *Otitis Media and Child Development.* Parkton, Md: York Press, 1986, pp 83-96.
13. Eimas PD, Clarkson RL: Speech perception in children: Are there effects of otitis media?, in Kavanagh JF (ed): *Otitis Media and Child Development.* Parkton, Md: York Press, 1986, pp 139-159.

Hearing Loss and Development: A Neuropsychologic Perspective

Cynthia Chase, PhD

Points To Recall:
- *Hearing loss in the first 3 years of life is associated with lower test scores for speech and language, cognitive ability, and school achievement.*
- *Children who experienced otitis media in the 1st year of life demonstrate behavior and attention differences compared to controls.*

Considerations for Referral:
- *Difficulty learning to read*
- *Distractibility, impulsiveness, or inattention*
- *Known hearing loss*

The challenge of early diagnosis of hearing loss in children, whether the degree of loss is mild, moderate, or severe, is a critical one. In the case of moderate or severe conductive or sensorineural loss, the guidelines for comprehensive diagnosis and remediation are clearer than they are in the case of mild hearing loss. In the case of mild hearing loss in a child, the pediatrician is faced with important management and referral decisions on the basis of evolving and sometimes conflicting research findings on the effects of mild hearing loss in childhood.

Hearing loss in infants, even moderate or severe in degree, is not easily detected in clinical practice. Detection requires vigilance, including routine identification of high-risk infants and adequate audiometric procedures. The average age at which sensorineural hearing loss is detected in children has been reported to be 1.5 to 2.5 years.[1]

Clinicians must be aware of the inadvisability of screening or not screening for hearing impairment on the basis of parental concern. In a recent study in Great Britain,[2] parents suspected the presence of hearing loss in only 44% of the children with severe or profound deafness. Parental suspicion was even lower for those with a mild or moderate permanent hearing loss. The advent of improved screening of high-risk infants has dramatically increased the percentage of hearing-impaired children identified in infancy.

The diagnosis of mild hearing loss should not be based on a cursory screening of language development; the child's use of words in isolation may be misleading. The assessment of language development in a child older than 2.5 years should include not only an assessment of how clearly the child speaks and the size of the child's vocabulary but also the length and complexity of phrases or sentences and the child's progress in developing proper syntax and morphology.

The older the child, the more subtle are the differences in language development due to mild hearing loss and the more difficult it is for the practicing pediatrician to detect abnormalities by listening to the child's spontaneous conversation. The spontaneous language of school-age children with mild hearing loss does not readily attract attention because their articulation, unlike that of children with more severe hearing loss, is usually adequate, and their sentence construction may not be strikingly unusual. However, when the more subtle aspects of language are formally assessed, school-age children with mild conductive hearing loss do show delays in vocabulary morphology (eg, with verb endings indicating tense) and difficulty with complex syntactic forms (eg, forming complex sentences).

Conductive Hearing Loss Due to Otitis Media

The most common cause of conductive hearing loss in children is otitis media. When a child has otitis media with effusion, the fluid in the ear frequently may persist for weeks or, in some children, for months, significantly impairing the child's hearing acuity. Using a behavioral test for hearing in infants, Huber et al[3] found that the presence of a conductive hearing loss in infants correctly predicted the presence of acute otitis media in 87% of cases.

Fluid in the middle ear reduces sound conduction by 25 dB on average. Although a child with a mild loss of approximately 25 dB is able to hear many sounds, he or she is apt to miss others. Softer speech sounds and voiceless consonants may be missed or confused when hearing loss is at a 10- to 20-dB level. A child may misunderstand and may be slower to appreciate the subtleties of language, such as verb tense, eg, *climbed* versus *climbing* and *sweep* versus *swept*, and comparatives such as *larger* and *largest*. It is also important to remember that, while the average loss is 25 dB with middle ear effusion (MEE), a certain percentage of children experience a greater hearing loss during periods of MEE and will miss a greater percentage of speech sounds. A 1984 policy statement of the American Academy of Pediatrics Committee on Early Childhood Adoption and Dependent Care[4] stated that

> There is growing evidence demonstrating a correlation between middle ear disease with hearing impairment and delays in the development of speech, language, and cognitive skills. When a child has frequent recurring acute otitis media and/or middle ear effusion persisting for longer than 3 months, hearing should be assessed and the development of communicative skills must be monitored.

Many investigators have concluded that such hearing impairments interfere with speech and language development, and some have described adverse effects on learning. Although a significant and persistent hearing loss in early childhood will undoubtedly lead to slower language and academic development, the long-term effects of a fluctuating and mild conductive hearing loss often associated with otitis media are more controversial. Various investigators have reported that children with a history of otitis media with effusion have deficits in verbal ability, lower verbal IQ scores than do children with no history of otitis media, and deficits in auditory processing.[5-9] Consistent with these findings, a positive history of otitis media and hearing loss is more common in populations of learning-disabled children than in their normally achieving peers.[9,10]

The Boston Otitis Media Studies

The results of a 7-year longitudinal study by the Greater Boston Otitis Media Study Group[11] support an association of recurrent otitis media during the first 3 years of life and lowered performance on tests of speech and language, intellectual, and academic skills at age 7 years. In this study, 207 children were randomly selected from a cohort of 498 and followed prospectively from birth until age 7 years. After confounding variables such as socioeconomic status and sex were controlled for, estimated time spent with MEE during the first 3 years of life was significantly associated with lower scores on tests of speech and language, cognitive ability, and school achievement.[11]

The Wechsler Intelligence Scale for Children-Revised (WISC-R) results from the Greater Boston Study are shown in Table 1. A clear relationship is seen between otitis media early in life and Full Scale IQ at age 7 years. The adjusted mean Full Scale WISC-R IQ was 113.1 for children with the least time, 107.5 for children with moderate time, and 105.4 for those with most time with MEE. Similar significant differences were found for Verbal and Performance IQs, indicating that both verbal and nonverbal skills were adversely affected by early otitis media and, presumably, early fluctuating hearing loss. Otitis media in the first 3 years was significantly associated also with lower scores in mathematics and reading. After time spent with MEE during the first 3 years of life was considered, time spent after age 3 years was not a significant predictor of IQ or achievement scores.

Table 1. Otitis Media in Infancy and Development of Speech, Language, and Cognitive Abilities in Boston Children Tested at Age 7 Years.[11] Results of Wechsler Intelligence Scale for Children-Revised.

	Time Spent With Middle Ear Effusion to Third Birthday		
	< 30 days N = 58	30-129 days N = 77	> 130 days N = 59
Full Scale IQ	113.1	107.5††	105.4***
Verbal IQ	111.5	106.5†	105.8**
Performance IQ	112.2	108.3	104.1***

< 30 days v >130 days: ***$P < 0.001$, **$P < 0.01$
< 30 days v 30-129 days: ††$P < 0.01$, †$P < 0.05$

What explains these results? How is it possible for both verbal and nonverbal skills to be affected by early fluctuating conductive hearing loss? There may be both a learned or behavioral and an organic basis to these findings. Animal studies have demonstrated that auditory deprivation early in the life of an animal can lead to detectable differences in brain development.[12] There is also evidence that severely hearing-impaired children demonstrate different patterns of brain organization than do children with normal hearing.[13] Evidence that auditory deprivation can cause differences in brain development is consistent with the hypothesis that not only speech and language but also other neuropsychologic functions, particularly attention, which has a pervasive role in learning and performance, may be affected by even mild and fluctuating hearing loss, such as that associated with otitis media.

To gain comprehensive understanding of the effects of early otitis media on children's learning style, it may be necessary to examine the full spectrum of cognitive functions. These include not only receptive and expressive language but also verbal and visual memory, construction, and graphomotor (drawing) and motor skills, as well as reading and writing. The central role of attention and concentration in relation to each of these cognitive functions is illustrated in the Figure.

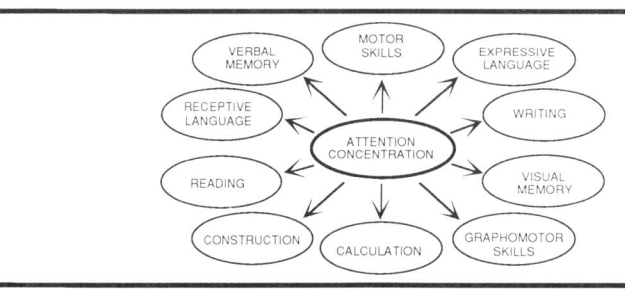

Figure. Neuropsychologic functions applicable to studies of otitis media.

In a study of otitis media in children from birth to 3 years of age by the Greater Boston Otitis Media Study Group [unpublished], a broader range of outcome variables is being analyzed to better our understanding of both 1) the earliest signs of developmental difficulty in children who demonstrate deficiencies as the result of their experience with otitis media and early temporary hearing loss and 2) mediating factors that are predictive of a benign outcome in children who have experienced recurrent otitis media and fluctuating hearing loss but show no deficits in later intellectual and academic skills.

Children were randomly selected from a study population of those with otitis media and drug prophylaxis to be seen for formal speech and language and neuropsychologic assessment at ages 1, 2, and 3 years. One hundred thirty-two children were followed from birth. The children were all from middle- or upper-middle-class homes in the Boston suburbs. Children were not seen when they were acutely ill. Cognitive and motor development was measured with the Bayley Scales of Infant Development. Questionnaires concerning the parents' perception of the children's usual health, temperament, and behavior were completed. In addition, each child's behavior was rated and analyzed, both during testing and during a structured interaction with the mother, in which the mother was asked to teach the child specific tasks.

Results at age 1 year, comparing children with varying frequencies of otitis media and those who did not have otitis media in the 1st year, are shown in Table 2. There were no differences between these groups in overall mental or motor development as measured by the Bayley Scales. However, there were clear behavioral differences between 1-year-old children who experienced recurrent otitis media in the 1st year and those who did not. Children who had experienced otitis media in the 1st year were rated as less attentive and less persistent by the examiner during testing and more irregular in their patterns of sleeping, eating, and elimination by their parents. In addition, children who had experienced otitis media were less responsive and less attentive when working with their mothers in a learning situation. These findings suggest that a child who has experienced ear infection and mild hearing loss may show signs of attentional difficulty very early in life.

Table 2. Otitis Media (OM) and Developmental Outcome at Age 1 Year.

Mental and motor development of children with OM
   No differences from disease-free controls in Bayley Mental or Motor scores due to OM
Behavior of children with OM
   Less attentive and persistent, as rated by examiner
   More irregular in sleeping, eating, elimination according to parents
   Less responsive in structured interaction with parent
Behavior of parents of children with OM
   Less skillful at providing effective teaching

Surprisingly, parents of children who had experienced otitis media were less effective teachers in the structured interaction. They were less effective in gaining the child's attention, less able to respond effectively when the child was distracted from the task, and less able to help the child understand and perform the task.

Guidelines for Clinical Practice

Data such as these broaden the scope of clinical concern. These findings suggest that another of the effects of otitis media and recurring mild conductive hearing loss, which may occur even in infancy, is interference with the child's attentional skills and with the quality of parent-child interaction.

Children with a history of persistent MEE and/or mild hearing loss need to be monitored carefully. Our current understanding suggests the following guidelines for clinical practice:

1) Parents of a child who is experiencing hearing loss, either temporary or permanent, often do not realize that the child has a hearing loss or that their communication with the child may be adversely affected by the child's hearing loss.

2) Parents should be instructed to a) establish face-to-face contact before speaking to the child, b) provide frequent feedback and cuing to the child as needed, c) be aware that a noisy environment makes it more difficult for the child to select and attend to what he or she needs to hear, d) speak slowly and clearly, and e) repeat if the child may not have heard what was said.

3) When a child in the early school years is experiencing difficulty in learning to read, the physician should consider whether the child has experienced hearing loss as the result of otitis media or other risk factors. Such a hearing impairment, even if resolved, may result in subtle lags in cognitive and speech and language development that predispose the child to difficulty with phonetic and reading skills.

4) The pediatrician seeing a distractible, impulsive, or inattentive child should keep in mind the possibility of hearing loss, either current or past, as a potential cause of the child's attentional problem.

5) Referral for neuropsychologic as well as careful linguistic assessment should be considered for children with a significant history of middle ear disease or diagnosis of hearing impairment.

References
1. Epstein S, Reilly JS: Sensorineural hearing loss. *Pediatr Clin North Am* 1989;36:1501.
2. Watkins PM, Baldwin M, Laoide S: Parental suspicion and identification of hearing impairment. *Arch Dis Child* 1990;65:846.
3. Huber C, Strangler S, Routh D: The BOEL test as a screening device for otitis media in infants. *Nurs Res* 1978;27:178.
4. American Academy of Pediatrics Committee on Early Childhood Adoption and Dependent Care Policy Statement: Middle ear disease and language development. *AAP News* 1984;35:9.

5. Zinkus PW, Gottlieb MI: Patterns of perceptual and academic deficits related to early chronic otitis media. *Pediatrics* 1980;66:246.
6. Schleiper A, Kisilevsky H, Mattingly S, et al: Mild conductive hearing loss and language development: A one year follow-up study. *J Dev Behav Pediatr* 1985;6:65.
7. Silva PA, Kirkland C, Simpson A, et al: Some developmental and behavioral problems associated with bilateral otitis media with effusion. *J Learn Disabil* 1982;15:417.
8. Silva PA, Chalmers D, Stewart I: Some audiological, psychological, educational and behavioral characteristics of children with bilateral otitis media with effusion. *J Learn Disabil* 1986;19:165.
9. Secord GJ, Erickson MT, Bush JP: Neuropsychological sequelae of otitis media in children and adolescents with learning disabilities. *J Pediatr Psychol* 1988;13:531.
10. Masters L, Marsh GE: Middle ear pathology as a factor in learning disabilities. *J Learn Disabil* 1978;11:103.
11. Teele DW, Klein JO, Chase C, et al: Otitis media in infancy and intellectual ability, school achievement, speech and language at 7 years. *J Infect Dis* 1990;162:685.
12. Webster DB: Conductive loss affects auditory neuronal soma size only during sensitive postnatal period, in Lim DJ, Bluestone CD, Klein JO, Nelson JD (eds): *Recent Advances in Otitis Media With Effusion*. Philadelphia: BC Decker, 1984, pp 344-346.
13. Woolf AB, Thatcher RW: Cortical reorganization in deaf children. *J Clin Exp Neuropsychol* 1990;12:209.

Language and Speech as a Management Guide and Outcome Measure

Robert J. Ruben, MD

Points To Recall:
- *Language delay can be caused by many biologic and/or social factors.*
- *Intervention for language delay must begin in the first 30 months of life.*
- *There are accurate diagnostic tests for many of the causes of language delay.*
- *There are effective interventions for many of the causes of language delay.*
- *Language is the outcome that is monitored in the care of communicative disorders.*

Considerations for Referral:
- *Failure of the Early Language Milestone screen*
- *Disproportionate levels of expressive and/or receptive language*
- *Failure of language to develop after intervention has commenced*

As we near the end of the 20th century, the development of optimal language is one of the most important missions of child health care. Language, heretofore, has not been considered the province of the physician, for there were the urgent needs of infectious disease in the domains of life, death, and function. As we have developed greater capacity to cure and care for life- or function-threatening infections, problems of communication and language disorders have become paramount. Deficits in the ability to communicate, ie, to have an effective language, hold substantial morbidity for the individual economically and socially and for society in its productivity and socialization.

The optimal development of language is based on the capacity of the central nervous system to receive the necessary input during the first 18 to 30 months of life. A multitude of diseases, disorders, and sociopathic conditions occur in infancy that adversely affect children's language. These include pathologies that have commonly been considered, such as hearing impairment, malformations of the voice-speech tract, and severe malformations or destruction of brain tissue. They also include conditions of the central nervous system that can adversely affect expressive or receptive language or an area of language such as semantics or syntax. There is the additional problem of auditory and language deprivation, which, in a severe form, has been documented in infants reared with minimal human contact. Other forms have been noted in children of mothers whose child-rearing knowledge and own language are so impoverished that their care of their children results in language deprivation.

The central nervous system appears to have a time-locked ability in the first 30 months of life to develop optimal language. The development of language is affected by a variety of conditions, including hearing impairment, specific neurologic disorders, and cultural deprivation. When two conditions are present, the patient appears to be more affected than would be expected from a sum of the two conditions. It is believed that these conditions are synergetic in the resulting language deficit.

Many pathologies that contribute to deficient language can be accurately diagnosed and there are effective interventions for the cure or care of these pathologies. The greatest difficulty has been to determine in a timely fashion which child has a high probability of a language deficit, since at least 10% of all children may have some form of language impairment.[1] Many attempts have been made to identify the children who are at risk for any one of the pathologies associated with language deficiency. Most of this work in infants has been done in the area of hearing screening. Overall, in western Europe and North America the results, for several reasons, have been unsatisfactory.[2] One important factor in the failure of these screening procedures has been that they have examined the cause and not the outcome of the disorder.

A pediatrician must have the methods to accurately and efficiently identify individual patients who are at risk for language deficit so that they may be evaluated. The use of the outcome, the language, to direct the management of the patient has been assessed and found to be effective.[3]

Early Language Milestone Scale

The Early Language Milestone (ELM) Scale developed and validated by Coplan[4,5] enables a physician, in a few minutes, to obtain an inventory of three aspects of an infant's language: expressive, receptive, and visual (Figure). The test is carried out in infants and toddlers from 1 to 38 months of age for language and to 47 months of age for speech. The parent is asked questions about the child's language and speech and/or the child is asked to carry out a few functions, eg, for receptive language, to identify what he or she drinks from. The combination of parental historic information, observational items, and results of simple tests are recorded on a form. The resulting matrix allows the physician to determine whether the child has passed or failed the ELM Scale. The

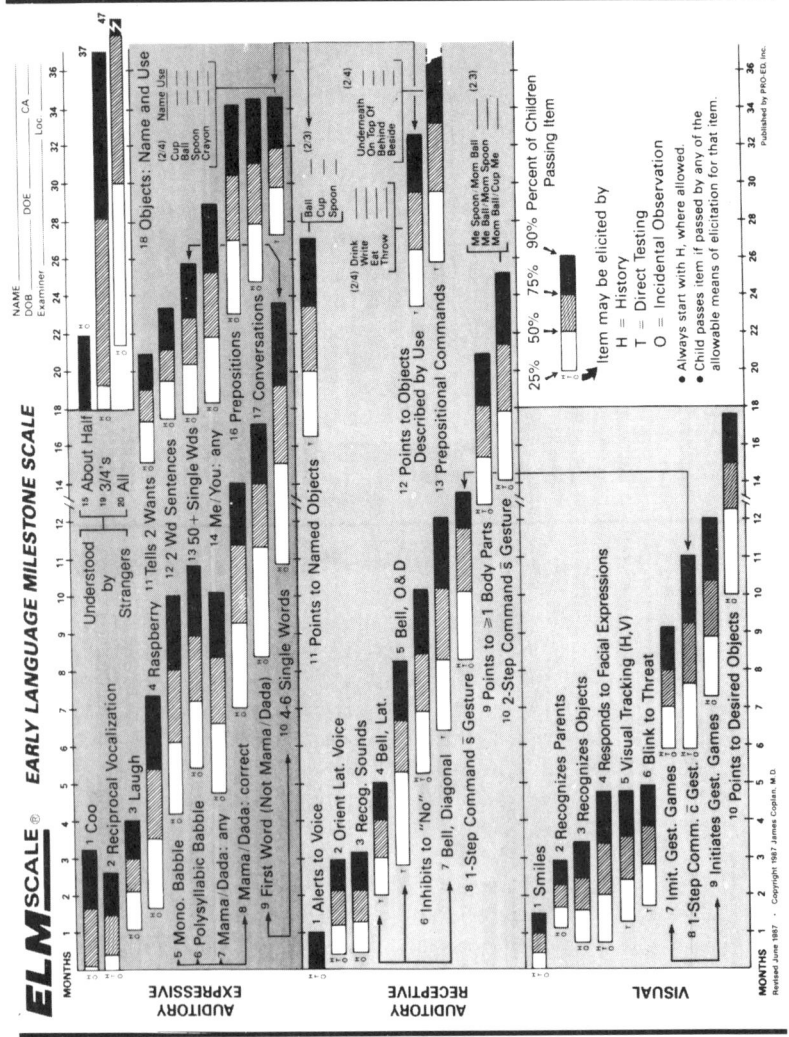

Figure. Early Language Milestone Scale (front). Reprinted by permission of James Coplan, MD.

Scale is devised to have a 10% failure rate. The sensitivity, specificity, and utility of the test have been found to be good.[3,6-10]

Experience at the Albert Einstein College of Medicine (AECOM) at the Montefiore Medical Center (MMC) with more than 500 patients has confirmed these reports and has found the ELM Scale to be efficient and effective. It is used by the Department of Otolaryngology in the following manner: Once the history and current illness have been elicited for a new patient, the ELM Scale is applied by the physician. While the interrogation and the observations are being carried out, other

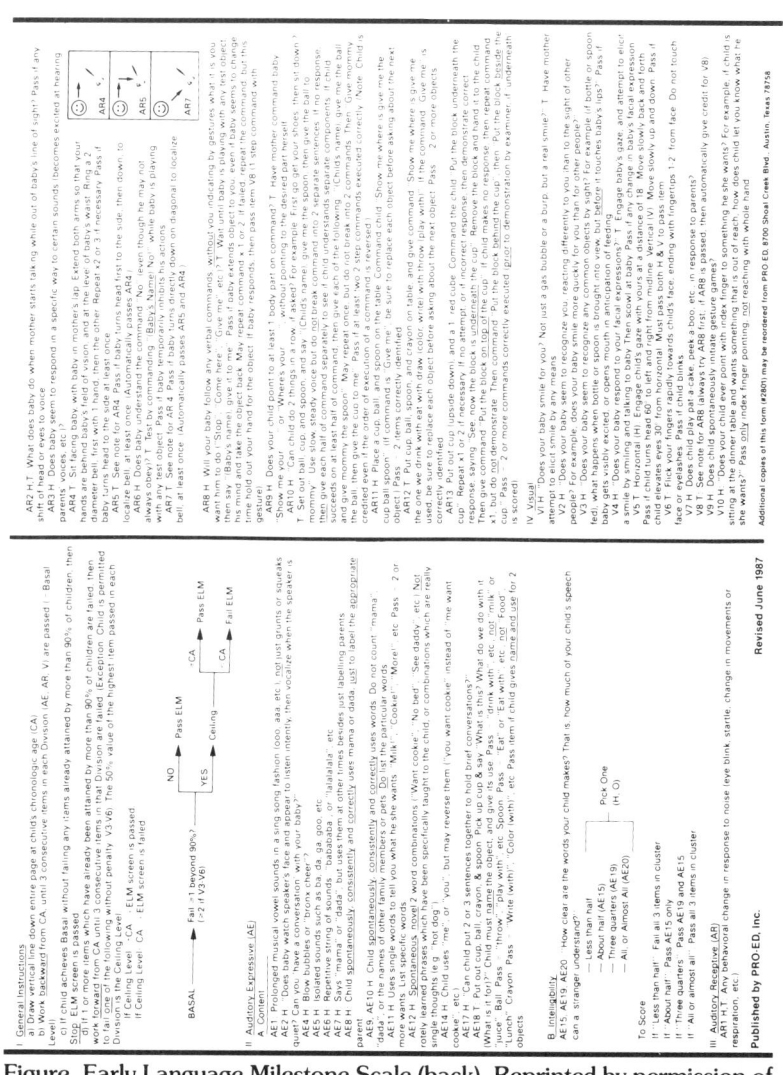

Figure. Early Language Milestone Scale (back). Reprinted by permission of James Coplan, MD.

useful information is often obtained. At the Department of Otolaryngology, only physicians have used the Scale, since it is believed that all aspects of the information are critical to the understanding of the complex problems of communication disorders. This policy is consistent with that of the physician always obtaining the entire medical history, and not having this done by another person, nor by having the patient fill out a form. Although the process is labor-intensive, it allows more information to be exchanged and encourages a closer bond between the physician and the patient and family.

The ELM Scale has been used consistently in all new patients younger than 3 years of age who have been seen in the pediatric otolaryngic practice of AECOM at MMC, and a review of 1 year's experience has been published.[3] The results of the ELM Scale are significant factors in determining the management of patients. The published data[3] reveal that the ELM Scale had a moderate to major effect in the management of about 30% of children (60/197). The definition of a moderate effect was "Results of the ELM were considered to contribute to the decision for implementation of an intervention"; for a major effect, the definition was "Results of the ELM contributed to the initiation of a major intervention such as an operation, the use of amplification, or enrollment in a habilitation program." Additionally, the results of the ELM Scale contributed to further evaluations in 36% of children (71/197). The number of children who need further management because of communication disorders is large in this practice, since it is a tertiary referral source specializing in communication disorders. The rate of failure for the ELM in a standard pediatric practice is approximately 10%.[4,7]

The information acquired from the ELM Scale is used in many ways. One frequent use is to make a management decision for a child with recurrent and/or persistent middle ear effusion (MEE). Further intervention will usually come about if the child has frequent febrile episodes, severe pathology of the tympanic membrane such as retraction or the beginning of incus necrosis, a hearing loss of 15 dB or greater in the speech frequencies in the better-hearing ear, and/or a language deficit. In 12- to 24-month-old children, hearing loss with MEE has been found to affect predominantly expressive language.[11,12]

Two case histories illustrate the way the ELM can be used: A 24-month-old child has had only a few febrile episodes secondary to otitis media. The physical examination reveals fluid behind the tympanic membrane but no retraction or other potentially serious change in the tympanic membrane. The child's hearing is between 10 and 15 dB in the speech frequencies. The tympanograms are "type B," or flat. The child has none of the conditions that are indicators for active intervention. Yet to be taken into account is the child's language level. If this child passes the ELM, he or she may be followed. If the child fails the ELM, especially in the expressive area, further management and evaluation will be undertaken.

Another child has a similar history but a 35-dB conductive hearing loss at the speech frequencies in the better-hearing ear. If the ELM

Scale is passed, the management will be directed at resolving the MEE, probably with antibiotics. The child will be periodically followed to ensure no further problems. If this child *fails* the ELM Scale, especially in the expressive area, there will be active therapy to improve the hearing, with either surgery or, in some special circumstances, amplification. The child will undergo detailed language and speech evaluations to determine the need for language training and/or other additional forms of habilitation.

The ELM Scale is also used to monitor progress and to evaluate effectiveness of intervention. Every 2 to 3 months, at least two types of data are obtained. First, hearing and middle ear status are evaluated. Heretofore, the outcome was considered successful if the child's hearing was normal. Second, the ELM Scale allows the physician to evaluate the child's language, which is the most critical outcome. If *language* has improved so that the child passes the ELM Scale, the intervention can be considered effective. However, if *hearing* is normal, there is no guarantee that language has developed appropriately. If the child should still fail the ELM Scale, further diagnostic procedures must be undertaken and/or interventions initiated.

As these examples show, the ELM Scale provides critical information for patient management. In the first instance, the physician is reassured that the hearing loss, which is mild when the child is seen, is not associated with the language deficit. This would suggest that the natural history of the interaction of the MEE, the hearing loss, and the language input in this particular child did not result in a language deficit. The physician can be conservative and follow the child. The child with a similar mild hearing loss who fails the ELM Scale may have a number of conditions that are not apparent at the time of examination. For example, the hearing may have been depressed at other times, or the day of the examination may have been the one day on which the child's hearing was normal. There may be other factors that, combined with the hearing loss, have resulted in the child's failing the ELM Scale. The failure alerts the physician to carry out further investigations to determine the extent, cause, and effective interventions for the language delay.

The ELM Scale has contributed to the management strategy in children with moderate hearing loss. Here again, the hearing is measured on what could be the worst day, the best day, or an average day. If a child passes the ELM, there is less reason for concern that the hearing loss may be a cause of or contributing factor to the language deficit. Management can then be directed toward the effusion and may not have to result in rapid restoration of hearing. On the other hand, a 24-month-old child with a 30-dB loss who fails the ELM Scale must be considered to have a high probability of a hearing loss as a cause of language delay. In this instance, interventions should be instituted promptly to restore the hearing and to improve language. The Scale is used to monitor the outcome of the interventions.

The ELM Scale was designed primarily to identify potential language abnormalities in children younger than 3 years of age, and the Scale does this well. A common problem is sensorineural hearing loss in children who are not diagnosed until 5 or 6 years of age. The all-too-common history is that the parents told the physician they were concerned about the slowness of the child's speech development but that they believed the child could hear. Parents seldom differentiate initially between speech and language, but do so after they have been given the definitions. Satisfactory hearing is thought to be demonstrated when the child responds to the jingling of keys or a noise-maker, and nothing more is done with regard to hearing. Many such children have been called "learning disabled" or "hyperactive" and/or have been given speech therapy. Hearing is finally evaluated in kindergarten or first grade, as a result of a failed screening test. The loss is identified, but too late for optimal language development and after emotional and social deprivation has occurred. The ELM Scale can detect these problems early, before the age of 3 years.

In another example, a 12-month-old child has not used "Mama/Dada" correctly and does not have a first word other than "Mama/Dada," cannot do a one-step command without a gesture, and cannot point to one or more body parts. This child would fail the ELM Scale at 12 months of age and would undergo further evaluations, including audiometric, speech and language, and neurologic, to determine if there is a language delay and, if so, its cause. The child might have a moderate sensorineural hearing loss that could be cared for with amplification and language habilitation, and then could be followed to determine if there was progression of the sensorineural loss.[13] The child would also have periodic ELM Scale ratings to determine if the interventions were effective in achieving the desired outcome of normal language.[14]

Although the examples here pertain to hearing loss, the ELM Scale has equal utility in other disorders resulting in language deficits. The Scale alerts the physician to language delay and results in modification of management to determine the cause and/or the effectiveness of various types of interventions that are used. The ELM Scale looks at language and speech as the outcome of a multitude of different diseases, disorders, and social conditions. It is like the stethoscope of the 19th century in that it notes abnormalities that must be defined. With the stethoscope, we were primarily concerned with asthma, pneumonia, and tuberculosis, all of which had similar outcomes as manifested by diversity of abnormalities of auscultation. We can now attend to hearing loss, language syndromes, social deprivation, and other neurologic disorders, all of which are manifested by the similar outcome of language delay.

References
1. Leske MC: Prevalence estimate of communication disorders in the United States. *ASHA* 1981;23:217.
2. Ruben RJ: Effectiveness and efficacy of early detection of hearing impairment in children. *Acta Otolaryngol Suppl* 1991;482:127.

3. Ruben RJ: Language screening as a factor in the management of the pediatric otolaryngic patient: Effectiveness and efficiency. *Arch Otolaryngol Head Neck Surg* 1991;117:1021.
4. Coplan J, Gleason J, Ryan R, et al: Validation of Early Language Milestone Scale in high-risk population. *Pediatrics* 1982;70:677.
5. Coplan J: *Early Language Milestone Scale.* Austin, Tex: PRO-ED Inc, 1983.
6. Coplan J, Gleason JR: Quantifying language development from birth to 3 years using the Early Language Milestone Scale. *Pediatrics* 1990;86:963.
7. Walker D, Gugenheim S, Downs MP, Northern JL: Early Language Milestone Scale and language screening of young children. *Pediatrics* 1989;83:284.
8. Black MM, Gerson LF, Freeland CA, et al: Language screening for infants prone to otitis media. *J Pediatr Psychol* 1988;13:423.
9. Satish M, McQuiston S, Dennler J, et al: Developmental testing I: Correlation of Early Language Milestone (ELM) at varying postnatal ages with Bayley. *Pediatr Res* 1988;23:455A.
10. Satish M, McQuiston S, Dennler J, et al: Developmental testing II: Correlation of multiple Early Language Milestone (ELM) with Bayley. *Pediatr Res* 1988;23:455A.
11. Wallace IF, Gravel JS, McCarton CM, Ruben RJ: Otitis media and language development at 1 year of age. *J Speech Hear Disord* 1988;53:245.
12. Wallace IF, Gravel JS: Otitis media and language development: A 2-year follow-up (abstract). New York: Society for Ear, Nose, and Throat Advances in Children Meeting Abstracts, 1988, p 28.
13. Ruben RJ, Fishman G: Otological care of the hearing impaired child, in Gerber S, Mencher G (eds): *Proceedings of Third Elks International Conference on Early Management of Hearing Loss.* New York: Grune & Stratton, 1980, pp 105-119.
14. Ruben RJ, Umano H, Silver M: Assessment of efficacy of intervention in hearing impaired children with speech and language deficits. *Laryngoscope* 1984;94:10.

Discussion

Dr Klein: Where are the gaps that need to be filled to make the case even more compelling that otitis media has a significant effect on speech/language and/or psychologic landmarks?

Dr Chase: I think what is missing is the longitudinal study that we and other researchers are attempting to do from very early in life until well into the school years. Further, we must look more closely at children's abilities and throw our nets wider to look at neuropsychologic functions, which include nonverbal skills, attentional skills, and speech and language skills.

Dr Feagans: Otitis media is a kind of "natural experiment," where the child experiences periods of deprivation, but we really don't know the total significance of those periods.

Dr Klein: So let's take it from the theoretic range and provide some guidance for pediatricians who have patients with chronic middle ear effusion. What should be recommended?

Dr Ruben: The ELM. But the ELM is a high fence, not a low fence. If a child fails the ELM, the pediatrician must look into the possibility of otitis media. If this is not responsible, the pediatrician can investigate another cause for language delay, such as sensorineural hearing loss.

Dr Eavey: In terms of the busy pediatrician in the community, is it possible to train someone in the office to do screening with the ELM?

Dr Ruben: I would think anybody could do it. I prefer to do it myself.

Dr de Villiers: Once we identify a child as having difficulty on a screening device like this, there are professionals who are trained to evaluate that language loss. I share some of the difficulties and skepticism that the primary physician may have about the range of variability because I think that we also have to make clear that, around the age of 2 years, there is a great deal of individual variability, a great deal of cultural variation in that early development.

According to the language data on otitis media, it is not really in the early single words that the difficulties are found. It's in the much more subtle aspects of language that have to do with functional words and small markings of meaning in the word and in complex sentences. Those turn out to be the factors that are predictive of good literacy development, which is why these children later have these kinds of reading problems.

Other factors influence language. One is that the early development of the ability of the child in narrative is closely related to early exposure to story-sharing. This is perhaps the strongest predictor of early reading and writing development.

Dr Brookhouser: Hearing loss is really a tremendous family stress factor, in terms of interaction between parent and child. We need to look more closely at what we know about undiscovered hearing losses and the vulnerability that some of these children have for abuse in dysfunctional families; some of the findings about cognitive deficits may well have a basis in other things than just otitis media.

Session V—
Management

Hearing Aids and Assistive Devices
Chris Halpin, PhD

Points To Recall:
- *Pediatric hearing testing and amplification should be referred to an audiologist.*
- *Possible hearing loss should be evaluated promptly in cases of parental concern or other risk factors.*
- *There is no audiologic reason to postpone testing, regardless of age; hearing aids can be fitted even in neonates.*
- *The parent is responsible for obtaining hearing aids.*
- *In school, consistent amplification relies on planning, acceptance, and monitoring.*
- *An FM trainer may be recommended for classroom use.*

Hearing aids are used to amplify sounds from normal volume to loud—in some cases, intensely loud—levels. Unlike with the eye, the specific deficiency of the ear is not corrected to a normal standard; the external sound environment is boosted electronically to a level that provides some degree of benefit to the listener. The expectations for benefit, therefore, are quite complex and depend primarily on the input capacity of the diseased ear. The evaluation of the input capacity of the ear in the normal sound environment and the comparable capacity in the amplified environment depend on precise clinical measurement and considerable experience. Patients needing pediatric hearing testing and amplification should be referred promptly to an audiologist, who will recommend further services by teachers of the hearing-impaired and other special educators.

Hearing aids can be used successfully for both conductive and sensorineural hearing loss. This paper discusses their use in pediatric patients with sensorineural hearing loss (SNHL). Four basic principles may be applied to the use of amplification for hearing-impaired children: Hearing aids should be applied quickly, precisely, flexibly, and consistently.

Applying Hearing Aids Quickly

Prompt amplification for a child depends on a referral from a pediatrician, neonatologist, or otolaryngologist to an audiologist to rule out hearing loss. This referral is recommended by the Joint Committee on Infant Hearing, based on a recently revised set of risk factors[1] [see

Appendix A]. Nearly 50% of children who need hearing aids will not present with the previously used set of risk factors.[2] Therefore, parental concern about hearing and language has been added as an official criterion in order to improve sensitivity. For most children who are referred, amplification will not be necessary, but this should not be cause to relax vigilance or to rely on less rigorous screening tests.

The consequence of delayed diagnosis is profound. Evidence includes a large longitudinal study by Markides,[3] who found that children who were identified with SNHL and who received amplification within the first 6 months showed far greater language development than did those who did not receive amplification until later. In short, the clock is ticking. Acquisition of language is a crucial task for young children, and hearing impairment should be diagnosed quickly.

Children can be tested and hearing aids can be used at any age. Newborns, for example, need a chance to listen and organize their auditory world for months before they speak. There are no audiologic reasons to postpone testing, and hearing aids, if indicated, must be fitted without delay. Grieving parents may feel that they should not act to remediate a confirmed loss until the cause is found, but while they are seeking alternate opinions about etiology, their child should be using hearing aids.

To fit hearing aids quickly, an audiologist must have the support of the child's primary physician. Most pediatricians will see children with hearing aids at some point, so a specific referral relationship should be established with an audiologist.

Applying Hearing Aids Precisely

The second basic principle is that the amplification must be precise. One of the most common problems is underamplification. Hearing loss is not uniform with regard to the ceiling or uncomfortable loudness level. In general, SNHL does not raise this ceiling at the same rate as it raises the threshold for soft sounds. Sounds that are very loud to people with normal hearing may be just as loud to a hearing-impaired child. There is no widely used measure of the loudness ceiling in very young children and, as a result, overly conservative hearing-aid settings are used in many cases.[4] The work of Kamm et al[5] can be applied to estimate the proper values.

The power range of a hearing aid is typically selected for use at medium- to high-volume settings. However, these levels are not always used by parents and other caregivers, for various reasons. For example, hearing aids are sold with a set of specifications based on performance in the adult ear, but the sound is more intense in the smaller infant ear. This effect has been demonstrated to be only about 4 to 6 dB.[6] However, before the publication of research showing the small size of this effect, larger values were suspected and overly conservative output limits were applied.

There is concern that the amplified sound itself will further damage the child. Humes and Bess[7] published a tutorial in which they examined this issue. They concluded that most hearing-aid strategies, as used in common practice, will not result in further damage. In an interesting sidelight, a longitudinal study by Markides[8] showed improvement in threshold as the previously deprived ear began to use sound through amplification.

In approximately 6% of SNHL cases, there also may be progressive hearing loss due to hereditary factors.[9] If the child does not receive regular audiologic evaluation, this further loss may go unnoticed and the effectiveness of the initial hearing-aid fitting will be reduced accordingly.

On the other side of the equation, the fact that a child has a hearing loss does not always mean that a hearing aid will solve the problem. For example, a hearing aid can block out some sounds simply by occluding the ear canal. This is known as insertion loss. The consequences of intentionally causing canal interference with residual normal hearing in certain frequencies in order to make pitches in other frequencies abnormally loud must be weighed carefully. Frequencies around 2000 Hz contribute the most useful information to the understanding of speech. If these frequencies are normal, amplification of other frequencies may produce poorer results for the patient than if unaided.

A case in point is that of the rising audiogram: Thresholds for lower pitches are down and thresholds for higher pitches are normal. There is clearly a significant hearing loss. The thresholds in the low frequencies often can be shown to be the result of the activation of the normal, high-frequency areas as the sound wave travels from the base to the apex of the cochlea.[10] Occluding the ear with a hearing aid to amplify low-frequency sound would interfere with usable high-frequency hearing.

The use of two hearing aids, while generally good practice, may also lead to unwanted results. In the case of two impaired ears, if one ear has a very asymmetric, distorted sound relative to the other, attempts to remediate both ears may lead to a competition that does not benefit the patient. In the case of one impaired and one normal-hearing ear, this same principle applies, so that, typically, no hearing aid is used. A thorough audiologic examination will reveal what is audible with a hearing aid, how and at what cost that audibility is achieved, and how the hearing aid is likely to affect development.

A child of any age can be tested with hearing aids in place to define precise amplification. The two major categories of such testing are functional-gain and real-ear measurement. Functional-gain testing is done by remeasuring the hearing with the hearing aids in place, using calibrated speakers in a sound booth. The child's reaction to hearing aids can be observed, and this sometimes results in better parental acceptance of the hearing aids.

Real-ear measurements are done with the hearing aid in place and a small, flexible tube alongside the aid in the ear canal. This probe tube permits sound to be measured within the ear canal itself. The output of the hearing aid can then be adjusted in situ to the target values selected by the audiologist. This is especially helpful, for example, when the expected normal resonance of the ear canal has been altered by surgery. As the normal ear canal grows, a complex and variable relationship with sound resonance occurs and can be measured. Real-ear measurement is not without its difficulties, however. It is sensitive to insertion depth and other factors, and it requires the quiet cooperation of the child. For precise amplification, the physician must evaluate the child's general physical and mental health and the health of the ear in particular, specifically noting the possibility of conditions such as cerumen impaction, otitis media, perforation, and otitis externa, and also considering the prognosis for progressive disease. The audiologist must evaluate the capacity of the ears and the benefit of the hearing aids. This basic cooperation, based on precise measurement and accumulated experience, will result in the maximum benefit for the patient.

Applying Hearing Aids Flexibly

The third basic principle is flexibility. For neonates, a body-worn type of hearing aid is often a good starter. Such a device has the broadest range of sound, is generally easy for parents to manipulate, and is well suited for the close, one-to-one communication typical at this age. At later ages, a behind-the-ear aid can be used with a series of ear molds. A feature that is clearly needed for flexibility is a direct audio connection, or "boot." With this plug, the child's individual aid conveys the output of another electronic device, such as a teacher's microphone or a television set.

Applying Hearing Aids Consistently

The fourth basic principle is to amplify consistently. Despite all the theoretic and technical difficulties associated with the other principles, this principle is the most difficult to enact. First, the parent is responsible for obtaining the hearing aids. If there is confusion or reluctance on the part of the parents, then physicians, audiologists, teachers, and others must consistently remind them of this responsibility. Hearing aids range in price from $300 to $1500 apiece, with an average near $800. The price generally excludes medical costs and initial audiologic testing. The cost is a great burden for some parents, but help is generally available through health departments and school systems. Each agency has its own rules, criteria, and reporting requirements; therefore, the assistance of a social worker or advocate should be enlisted early in the process. The cost in time includes one to three visits for specific hearing-aid evaluation and the taking of ear-mold impressions, another one to three visits for fitting and testing, and periodic rechecks ranging from one per month to an annual visit for maintenance. Generally, younger infants require the most time at each stage.[11] The child must also have clear responsibilities. By the age of 5 years, the child should be able to put the aid in and take it out, alert the parents to dead batteries, change batteries, and even help order replacements.

In school, consistent amplification relies on planning, acceptance, and monitoring. The use of the hearing aids must be clearly stated in the child's individual education plan. School administrators, parents, and teachers must work together to nip in the bud any negative reactions by teachers or students. A consistent monitoring program must be clearly stated, documented, and reviewed by an effective teacher or administrator.[12]

Assistive Listening Devices

Assistive listening devices (ALDs) consist of the same basic audio components as hearing aids and are also personally fitted to the user. The difference, which is of critical importance to the pediatric patient, is the source of the sound. In an ALD, the sound does not originate from a microphone at the patient's ear but from a microphone worn by the speaker. This microphone placement reduces the harmful interference of room noise and enhances the informative signal. Such an improvement in the signal-to-noise ratio has been shown to be the most effective electronic enhancement for SNHL.[13] One of the more common examples of this device is called the FM trainer because the signal is transmitted from the teacher to the student by FM radio. In cases of severe hearing loss, this strategy is so beneficial that the FM unit may be recommended as the child's first hearing aid, with the more general hearing aid added later. If the FM trainer is intended for use in the classroom, the school system usually accepts the responsibility for purchase and maintenance.[14] Auditoriums and churches are increasing their use of this strategy for providing the hearing-impaired person with the signal directly. Such broadcast systems use FM radio, electromagnetic field, or infrared light.

Other Devices

A number of other devices are useful to hearing-impaired patients and their parents. These involve the use of other senses in creative ways. For example, there are devices that cause a light to flash when the doorbell rings, an alarm clock that vigorously vibrates under the pillow, and closed-caption TV, in which the printed text of a program is seen at the bottom of the screen. A very helpful device for the severely hearing-impaired is the Telecommunications Device for the Deaf (TDD). Two persons who have TDDs can communicate by telephone. Some communities have relay centers where an operator with a TDD can voice the messages of a caller to other parties who have voice phones only.

Common Problems

Pediatricians may hear complaints and questions from parents about the common problems associated with hearing aids and assistive devices.

Feedback, an annoying whistling sound, is caused when sound from the hearing-aid output leaks out and is recaptured by the microphone. This causes a chain reaction that quickly develops into a characteristic squeal. Leaks are easily formed in the soft pinnae of young children and are to be expected as the ear grows while the ear mold does not. In most cases, patients aged 0 to 5 years will need two ear molds per year, those aged 6 to 12 years will need one per year, and adolescents will need one every 2 years.[15] Even when the ear mold fits perfectly, placing a reflective surface, such as a blanket, in proximity to the hearing aid can cause sound to be reflected into the microphone. When feedback occurs, correct remedial action is to reseat the ear mold, get a new ear mold, or remove the reflective surface. However, the remedial action often taken by the parent is to turn the hearing-aid volume down until the whistling stops. This is a persistent cause of underamplification.

Other issues can arise. Otitis media with perforation and active drainage is often a temporary contraindication for hearing-aid use.[16] In the more common case, where an intact drum is present, the aid may continue to be worn. Hearing aids tend to last 3 to 5 years with normal use, but pediatric patients often lose the aids, immerse them in water, feed them to the dog, etc. There are several helpful products for young children that snug the aids to the ears and prevent loss. Parents would also be well advised to insure the aids against loss and damage. Parents should be clearly informed of the extremely serious nature of the ingestion of batteries by young hearing-aid users, and the appropriate poison referral number should be attached to the telephone and explained to all who care for the child. Finally, many parents cling to high expectations for "fixing" the problem. This may stem, in part, from experience with the total correction often available with eyeglasses. The situation is more analogous to fitting eyeglasses on a patient with a degenerated retina. The input channel is severely limited and it is that limitation, more than any other factor, that governs the benefit expected from hearing aids.

References

1. Joint Committee on Infant Hearing: 1990 position statement. *AAO-HNS Bull* 1991;10:15.
2. Stein L, Clark S, Kraus N: The hearing impaired infant: Patterns of identification and habilitation. *Ear Hear* 1983;4:232.
3. Markides A: Age at fitting of hearing aids and speech intelligibility. *Br J Audiol* 1986;20:165.
4. Kawell M, Kopun J, Stelmachowitz P: Loudness discomfort levels in children. *Ear Hear* 1988;9:133.
5. Kamm C, Dirks D, Mickey M: Effect of sensorineural hearing loss on loudness discomfort level and most comfortable loudness judgments. *J Speech Hear Res* 1978;21:668.
6. Feigin J, Kopun J, Stelmachowitz P, Gorga M: Probe tube microphone measures of ear canal sound pressure levels in infants and children. *Ear Hear* 1989;10:254.
7. Humes L, Bess F: Tutorial on the potential deterioration in hearing due to hearing aid usage. *J Speech Hear Res* 1981;46:3.

8. Markides A: The use of individual hearing aids by hearing impaired children: A long term survey, 1977-1987. *Br J Audiol* 1989;23:123.
9. Parving A: Longitudinal study of hearing-disabled children: A follow-up investigation. *Int J Pediatr Otorhinolaryngol* 1988;15:233.
10. Thornton A, Abbas P: Low frequency hearing loss: Perception of filtered speech, psychophysical tuning curves and masking. *J Acoust Soc Am* 1980;67:638.
11. Martin F, Gravel K: Pediatric audiologic practices in the United States. *Hear J* 1989;42(8):33.
12. English K: Best practices in educational audiology. *Lang Speech Hear Serv Schools* 1991;22:283.
13. Plomp R: Auditory handicap of hearing impairment and the limited benefit of hearing aids. *J Acoust Soc Am* 1978;63:533.
14. Reichman J, Healy W: Amplification monitoring and maintenance in schools. *ASHA* 1989;30(11):43.
15. Sweetow W: Fitting forum: ITE's for children revisited, 1990. *Hear Instruments* 1990;41(8):40.
16. Alvord L, Doxey G, Smith D: Hearing aids worn with tympanic membrane perforation: Complications and solutions. *Am J Otol* 1989;10:277.

Cochlear Implants in Children
William M. Luxford, MD

Points To Recall:
- *A multichannel cochlear implant has been approved by the FDA for use in children.*
- *Cochlear implants in children are* not *experimental.*
- *Cochlear implants are not hearing aids.*
- *Candidates have profound, bilateral sensorineural hearing loss and do not benefit from conventional amplification.*
- *Surgical and postoperative complications have been minimal.*
- *Implants increase auditory abilities and improve speech-production skills.*
- *Although postlingually deafened children in oral programs as a group demonstrate the fastest and greatest development of auditory skills, congenitally and prelingually deafened children show substantial benefit.*

In recent years, the cochlear implant has become an acceptable alternative device beyond the hearing aid for providing auditory stimulation to people who are profoundly deaf. Two types of devices, a single-channel cochlear implant and a multichannel cochlear implant, have been used in investigational studies approved by the US Food and Drug Administration for children as young as 2 years of age. The Children's Center of the House Ear Institute has had considerable experience with the single-channel cochlear implant in the last 10 years and with the multichannel cochlear implant in the last 4 years.[1] In June 1990, following 4 years of clinical investigation for safety and efficacy in children, the FDA granted approval for clinical distribution of the multichannel implant in children. This device is the only implant system to have gained market-approval status for use in children. With this FDA approval, the procedure is no longer considered "investigational" or "experimental."

Components

The basic components of a cochlear implant are a microphone, signal processor, external transmitter, internal receiver/stimulator, and electrode array. In the multichannel cochlear implant, sounds are received by the directional microphone and routed to the speech processor. The speech processor amplifies, filters, and digitizes these signals and then selects and codes the elements of sound that are most useful for understanding speech. These electronic codes are sent to the internal receiver/stimulator via the external transmitter. The stimulator delivers electrical impulses to the appropriate electrodes in the cochlea. Each of the 22 electrodes is programmed separately to deliver signals that can vary in loudness and pitch. These electrodes then stimulate different hearing-nerve fibers, which send the messages on to the brain.

Candidates

Criteria for candidacy follow comprehensive selection guidelines as defined by the FDA investigation and by clinical experience with the device[1] (Table). The primary criterion for selection is confirmation of profound sensorineural hearing loss. Tympanometry and otoscopy are performed to rule out middle ear pathology at the time of testing.

Table. Candidate-Selection Guidelines for Cochlear Implants in Children.

Age 2 to 17 years
Profound, bilateral sensorineural hearing loss
No significant benefit with the use of conventional hearing-aid amplification
No medical or radiologic contraindications
Families and candidates (if age-appropriate) who have realistic expectations about potential benefits
Educational program that emphasizes development of auditory skills
Families and candidates well motivated to follow through with program aimed at maximizing the benefits of implantation

A child who is a candidate for an implant demonstrates poorer performance on selected auditory discrimination tasks while using appropriately fitted, powerful hearing aids than would be expected from children with implants. A cochlear implant is *not* a hearing aid. An implant can provide useful hearing for some children with profound hearing loss who do not benefit from traditional hearing or vibrotactile aids. Parent and teacher reports of the child's auditory ability should be consistent with the measured severity of the hearing loss. If recent hearing aids or ear molds have not been optimal and there is evidence of some usable residual hearing, a 3- to 6-month trial using appropriate aids and molds is required.

The medical evaluation includes a complete history and physical examination to detect problems that might interfere with the patient's ability to complete either the surgery or rehabilitation procedures. It is important to identify any external or middle ear disease, including perforations of the tympanic membrane, that must be treated before cochlear implantation.

High-resolution computed tomography of the temporal bone is performed preoperatively to identify partial or complete ossification of the scala tympani of the cochlea, soft-tissue obliteration of the scala, congenital malformation of the inner ear, and surgical landmarks. Complete agenesis of the cochlea and an abnormal acoustic nerve—the result of either congenital malformation, trauma, or surgery—are contraindications for cochlear-implant placement. Cochlear hypoplasia (Mondini deformity) is not a contraindication; children with such a malformation can use the multichannel implant successfully. Magnetic resonance imaging (MRI) is not practical for evaluating implant candidates, since MRI shows little bony detail and, as yet, not enough of the membranous inner ear. With future improvements, it may become more useful in detecting cochlear fibrosis. Ossification or fibrous occlusion of the cochlea or the round window does not preclude a cochlear implant, but it may influence the patient's response to implant stimulation. Parents and patients are counseled accordingly.

The evaluation process is designed to ensure that the family and, if possible, the child have realistic expectations about the potential benefits of a cochlear implant. The therapy and educational program in which the child is enrolled are vitally important. Therapists and teachers, in conjunction with the parents and audiologists, need to provide the child with appropriate listening models and materials for development of auditory skills.

Finally, the child's and family's motivation and commitment are critical to the child's ultimate adjustment to and benefit from the implant. The child must be willing to wear the device regularly and the family must be dedicated to keeping appointments, maintaining the device, and helping the child transfer listening skills to everyday situations.

Surgery

A cochlear implantation should be performed only by a qualified surgeon specifically trained in the procedure by the manufacturer of the implant. The implant is placed according to conventional surgical techniques developed to treat chronic middle ear disease. The surgical approach through the mastoid and facial nerve recess leaves the ear canal wall intact and provides direct access to the cochlear scala tympani. Placement of the implant in a child is essentially the same as in an adult, because the key anatomic structures, including the cochlea and ossicles, are in place and in their adult configurations at birth. By age 2 years, the mastoid antrum and facial nerve recess are adequately developed. Surgery to implant the internal receiver/stimulator takes approximately 2 to 3 hours under general anesthesia. The hospital stay is generally 1 or 2 days.

Risks

The risks of the implant procedure are the same as those for chronic ear surgery. These include infection, facial paralysis, cerebral spinal fluid drainage, meningitis, and the usual risks of anesthesia. Fortunately, the complications encountered by recipients of both the single-channel and multichannel implants (> 300 and > 400, respectively) have been exceptionally minimal. One concern about extending the cochlear-implant program to children was the risk of increased incidence or severity of otitis media, but information from clinical trials with both devices[1] revealed no increase in either incidence or severity of otitis media in children receiving the cochlear implants.

Device Fitting

Although most patients resume their normal activities within the 1st week following surgery, it takes 3 to 5 weeks for the incision to heal completely. After the healing process has occurred, the child returns to the clinic for the initial programming of the speech processor of the multichannel implant. An audiologist sets the appropriate levels of stimulation for each electrode, from soft to comfortably loud. Usually this process takes a few sessions. The parents participate actively during the lessons, which helps them realize the benefits and limitations of the implant and provides them with practice for working with the child at home. Following the initial stimulation period, the child goes back to his or her regular academic and therapy settings. The implant staff maintains contact with the school, providing information about the cochlear implant to teachers and therapists and offering suggestions on how to proceed with therapy.

Results

Considerable experience with cochlear implants has demonstrated that these devices can provide significant benefit to profoundly deaf children. Besides making the patient aware of environmental sounds, an implant can enable such children to detect much of the acoustic speech signal and to make stress and pattern discriminations. Many of these children can discriminate between spondees (words of two syllables with equal stress, eg, *baseball, cowboy*) in closed sets (ie, multiple choice) and can obtain nonzero scores on tasks requiring the open-set (auditory input only;

no choices) recognition of words and sentences. These auditory abilities are reflected in the development of improved speech-production skills.

Few tests are available that are appropriate for children of all ages and all levels of speech and language skill. Therefore, it is difficult to assess the performance of children with cochlear implants as a group, given their broad range of ages and language skills. Further, although group data are helpful for defining overall device-performance limits, it is difficult to make appropriate predictions and counsel effectively for an individual implant candidate. The definition of success differs from patient to patient and family to family. Several factors appear to affect the benefit a child may receive from an implant. Auditory memory appears to be one of the most important factors. Children who have had some auditory experience and a short period of deafness may learn to use the sound information provided by the implant more quickly and effectively than children who were born with profound hearing loss or lost their hearing very early in life.

Many professionals are concerned about whether congenitally deaf children can benefit from these devices, whether children in total-communication (using sign language also) educational programs can benefit, and whether children with cochlear implants are likely to receive the kind of training that will maximize the use of the implants. Experience with both implant devices indicates that, in fact, congenitally deaf children do show significant benefits from the implant, as do children in total-communication programs. However, just as with hearing aids, auditory skills are not likely to be maximized without appropriate auditory training.[1-3]

Availability

At present, the multichannel device is the only cochlear implant that is available for children; the single-channel device is no longer being manufactured. Like any sophisticated medical device, cochlear implants are expensive. Costs for preimplant evaluation, the implant system, surgery, and postsurgical fitting and training generally exceed $30,000. Because the FDA has approved the use of the multichannel cochlear implant in children, many insurance carriers (Blue Cross/Blue Shield, Medicaid, some HMOs, and most private insurance companies) will provide full or partial coverage.

The internal components of the multichannel implant are designed to last a patient's lifetime. However, as with any manufactured device, there is some risk of failure. In the unlikely event that an internal component fails, the cochlear implant can almost always be successfully replaced. Repair or replacement of the external components (microphone, cables, and speech processor) is needed much more often. The implant system is designed so that changes can be made in the external components or, if need be, the internal receiver/stimulator and electrode array can be replaced with a technologically superior system.

References

1. Berliner KI, Luxford WM, House WF: Cochlear implants in children, in Myers EN, Bluestone CD, Brackmann DE, Krause CJ (eds): *Advances in Otolaryngology—Head and Neck Surgery*. St Louis: Mosby Year Book Inc, 1990, pp 61-79.
2. Waltzman S, Cohen NL, Spivak L, et al: Improvement in speech perception and production abilities in children using a multichannel cochlear implant. *Laryngoscope* 1990;100:240.
3. Tonokawa LL, Luxford WM: Current results with multichannel cochlear implants in children, in press.

Discussion

Ms Tucker: I am curious to know if any studies have ever related the cause of deafness to the success of an implant.

Dr Luxford: Since meningitis is the most common cause for the patients who have received implants and this is an acquired loss, that's the largest group. For the other groups, the total numbers are too small. However, the likelihood is that a patient will do better after *H influenzae* meningitis than after pneumococcal meningitis due to destruction by bone growth within the cochlea.

Dr Thornton: One of our beliefs is that the number of nerve fibers that remain to be stimulated, at least theoretically, ought to have a relation with how well an implant can function. Nadol et al have shown that etiology does have a fairly good correlation with surviving nerve fibers [*Ann Otol Rhinol Laryngol* 1989;98:411].

Dr Luxford: Linthicum, however, when histologically studying patients who had already received implants and who had died from other causes, found no correlation with the number of remaining ganglion cells and function [Linthicum et al, *Am J Otol* 1991;12:245].

Mr Gjerdingen: Every bit of hearing helps. For example, a 6-dB difference doesn't sound like much, but we need to remember that 6 dB doubles the level of intensity. Therefore, a hearing aid or assistive device truly can provide benefit.

Dr Ruben: Pediatricians and family physicians should be aware that no infant or child is too young or too damaged for hearing measurement and some form of therapy.

Dr Hammerschlag: I would like to add that a referral for a hearing-aid evaluation and fitting obviously has to include aural rehabilitation, which takes a lot of time and practice.

Mr Gjerdingen: When choosing an audiologist to provide amplification for children, one must be sure that the audiologist is licensed, certified, and experienced in working with children.

Dr Klein: Considering the incidence of bacterial meningitis and the proportion of cases of sensorineural hearing loss that occur, we now have an effective *Haemophilus* vaccine at 2 months of age and anticipate pneumococcal and meningococcal vaccines. If these are successful, they should be able to prevent many cases of hearing loss.

Pediatricians need to be advocates for use of the vaccine at local, state, and federal levels and they also need to become advocates for the necessary funding.

Intervention Strategies for the Child With Recurrent or Persistent Middle Ear Disease

Stephen I. Pelton, MD

Point To Recall:
- *Recurrent otitis media and persistent middle ear effusion (MEE) are chronic illnesses of childhood.*

Considerations for Referral:
- *Patients with recurrent otitis and/or persistent effusion should be referred for audiology to determine the extent of hearing loss.*
- *Children who fail initial strategies for prevention of recurrent otitis or management of persistent MEE should have consultation with an otorhinolaryngologist, and a joint management program by pediatrician and ENT should be developed.*

The goals of medical management for children with recurrent or persistent middle ear disease include early identification of the child at risk, short-term strategies to prevent recurrences of acute otitis media and enhance the resolution of persistent middle ear effusion, and, finally, long-term strategies that reduce the burden of middle ear disease over an extended period. Each strategy requires careful consideration of the risks and benefits for an individual child. Two concepts must continually remain at the forefront of consideration for all interventions. First, none of the intervention strategies are curative but seek to prevent the disease and associated morbidity until the child "outgrows" this illness. Second, decisions regarding the initiation of therapy or medical versus surgical approaches require individualized considerations such as the extent of hearing loss, stage of language development, and participation in day care.

Middle ear disease in childhood may manifest itself as either recurrent episodes of acute otitis media or persistent MEE, or a combination of these events. Recurrent otitis media is predominantly a disease of early childhood. Studies by my colleagues in Boston[1] revealed that 17% of children in their 1st year of life had three or more episodes of otitis media. They observed that with each subsequent year, the percent of children suffering three episodes declined. In year 7 of life, only 3% of children were observed to have three or more acute episodes of otitis media. Similarly, persistent MEE is also observed most frequently in early infancy. We observed that children younger than 2 years of age were much more likely to have persistent effusion for more than 1 month after an acute episode than were children older than 2 years of age.[2] Each of these aspects of middle ear disease in childhood—acute recurrences and prolonged effusion following acute episodes—may require separate intervention strategies.

Several risk factors distinguish the child likely to suffer the greatest burden of middle ear disease [see Klein, this publication]. Studies by Teele and colleagues[1] and Marchant and colleagues[3] identified early onset of disease as an important predictor of an increased burden of middle ear disease. Children with a combination of these factors should be considered at high risk for middle ear disease, and intervention strategies should be proposed early, before the morbidity associated with multiple episodes of otitis or prolonged persistent effusion has occurred.

Prevention of Recurrent Otitis Media

Numerous trials of antimicrobial prophylaxis for the prevention of recurrent acute otitis media have demonstrated efficacy when administered over a limited period, most often 3 to 6 months. Recently, Principi et al[4] demonstrated a reduction in the number of acute episodes of otitis media in children on trimethoprim-sulfamethoxazole or amoxicillin prophylaxis given once daily. Sixty-three percent of the children receiving placebo had a recurrent episode during the 6th-month follow-up, compared to 27% of the children on prophylaxis with either agent. In our studies,[5] we observed a significant reduction in the number of episodes of acute otitis media as well as in the number of children suffering two or more episodes of otitis media among those given once-daily amoxicillin prophylaxis over a 6-month period. The spectrum of antimicrobial agents effective in preventing occurrences appears to be similar to the spectrum of antimicrobial agents effective for the therapy of acute otitis media, although not all antimicrobial agents have been studied. Results with each of the antimicrobial agents that have been evaluated appear comparable, and decisions regarding the selection of an antimicrobial agent for prophylaxis should focus on safety and cost. Current practice suggests that once-daily amoxicillin (20 mg/kg) or twice-daily sulfisoxazole (50 mg/kg per dose) is safe and is associated with good patient compliance.

Recent studies have demonstrated the limitations of antimicrobial prophylaxis for recurrent otitis media. Principi[4] demonstrated that even in children in whom antimicrobial prophylaxis for the prevention of recurrent episodes was effective, the proportion of time spent with MEE was large. Children in whom antimicrobial prophylaxis effectively prevented recurrences did have a small reduction in the proportion of time spent with middle ear disease compared with children who continued to have recurrent episodes; however, even these children spent a significant part of the 6-month follow-up with MEE.

In our studies,[5] we demonstrated a significant short-term benefit for children on antimicrobial prophylaxis. However, when the burden of recurrent otitis media in the placebo and antimicrobial-treated groups was evaluated over a 12-month period, little if any difference in the number of recurrent episodes was observed.

Both of these studies suggest limitations in the efficacy of prophylaxis with antimicrobial agents. Recurrent disease can clearly be prevented over a limited period, but persistent MEE and its associated hearing loss may persist. In addition, no "carry-over" benefit for prophylaxis was observed. It appears that once antimicrobial prophylaxis is discontinued, many high-risk infants will have recurrent episodes of otitis media.

Intervention Strategies for Persistent MEE

The pathophysiology that results in persistent MEE remains multifactorial. Microbiologic studies of children with persistent effusion demonstrate potential bacterial pathogens in as many as one third of children. Inflammatory mediators, such as prostaglandins and cytokines, have also been identified in MEEs in children at the time of tympanostomy-tube insertion, suggesting that ongoing inflammation is an important contributor to persistent effusion. These observations have led to the evaluation of antimicrobial and anti-inflammatory therapies in children with persistent effusion.

Healy[6] demonstrated that administration of trimethoprim-sulfamethoxazole daily over a 30-day period resulted in a greater proportion of children with effusion-free middle ears at follow-up than in children observed without any intervention strategy. This observation has been confirmed by Giebink and colleagues.[7]

The experience with anti-inflammatory agents has been much less consistent, and conflicting results have been observed. Several investigators[7,8] have demonstrated enhanced resolution of MEE in children treated with prednisone compared with those who received no treatment. Other investigators failed to demonstrate enhanced resolution of persistent MEE with oral dexamethasone.[9] Differences in results may be related to definitions of disease at entry as well as to the selection of specific anti-inflammatory agents such as prednisone versus dexamethasone.

Lastly, combinations of antimicrobial agents with anti-inflammatory agents have recently been evaluated. Berman et al[8] reported resolution of persistent MEE in 77% of patients treated with a combination of trimethoprim-sulfamethoxazole and prednisone compared to 30% in patients treated with trimethoprim-sulfamethoxazole alone. This area of investigation appears to have great potential and requires further evaluation. Unfortunately, even though short-term interventions that hasten the resolution of MEE have been demonstrated, a significant percentage of children develop acute otitis media within a short period after the resolution of effusion and, over a more extended period, have a recurrence of effusion that eventually necessitates tympanostomy-tube placement. Berman et al reported that 18% of children with complete resolution of effusion following treatment with trimethoprim-sulfamethoxazole and prednisone required insertion of tympanostomy tubes within 12 months.

Office Management of Children With Recurrent Middle Ear Disease

Children who present with otitis media in the first 6 months of life should be considered candidates for prophylaxis following the initial episode, if other risk factors are present. A child whose family has a history of recurrent or persistent middle ear disease, who attends group day care, and/or who has disease that begins in the fall or winter during respiratory-virus season should be considered for antimicrobial prophylaxis after only a single episode. In children in whom risk factors are not present, prophylaxis may not be necessary unless a second episode occurs before the child's first birthday. In children who have escaped disease during the 1st year of life, recurrent otitis media is less frequent. In these children, antimicrobial prophylaxis is not warranted for recurrent disease until two episodes have occurred within a 3- to 4-month period, or three episodes within a year. Currently, we choose amoxicillin (20 mg/kg per day given as a single dose) as initial therapy. There is no precise guideline for how long to continue antimicrobial prophylaxis if it is effective. Our experience suggests that once prophylaxis is discontinued, these children remain at high risk for additional episodes of acute otitis. I would continue prophylaxis throughout the respiratory-virus season, for a minimum of 3 months and a maximum of 6 months. During that period, it is necessary for the child to be evaluated regularly for the presence of MEE and its associated hearing loss.

If a child continues to be free of acute episodes and free of MEE, discontinuing therapy and continuing observation seem appropriate. After therapy is discontinued, if the child has an additional episode of acute otitis media, prophylaxis should be reinstituted after therapy for the acute episode is completed. Again, the child can be maintained on prophylaxis for 6 months, if effective. A child who has breakthrough episodes while on prophylaxis should be treated with an antimicrobial agent that has activity against the three most common pathogens, *Haemophilus influenzae*, *Streptococcus pneumoniae*, and *Moraxella catarrhalis*. An agent that is effective against both β-lactamase-producing and non-β-lactamase-producing isolates is most appropriate. For the child who has a second breakthrough of acute otitis media, alternative antimicrobial agents for prophylaxis should be considered. Limited studies are available to guide specific selection; however, antimicrobial agents effective against a broad spectrum of respiratory pathogens and used for acute otitis media are appropriate candidates for prophylaxis. Safety is a primary concern in considering trimethoprim-sulfamethoxazole, amoxicillin-clavulanate, ceclor, cefixime, or erythromycin-sulfisoxazole. No clearly superior agent is available, and decisions should be individualized after discussions with the parents about risks and benefits.

A child with persistent effusion also presents a difficult issue when defining precisely when to intervene. Natural-history studies[1,2] demonstrate that effusion persists after acute otitis in 40% of children at 1 month, 20% of children at 2 months, and 10% of children at 3 months. These studies suggest that persistent effusion resolves spontaneously each month in half of the children, and therefore it is not until after 3 months or more with persistent effusion that the likelihood of spontaneous resolution is small. Again, I focus on young children, who are more likely to have persistent effusion following acute otitis media. Unfortunately, it is just these children in whom quantifying the hearing loss associated with persistent effusion is difficult, requires auditory brainstem response (ABR) studies, and therefore cannot be done repeatedly. In addition, because of the variability in speech development in early infancy, it is difficult to determine which children are "delayed."

Intervention should be considered for the child whose persistent effusion has lasted more than 6 to 8 weeks after an initial episode of acute disease. The initial intervention would consist of a 1-month course of trimethoprim-sulfamethoxazole, given at 8 mg/kg per day in two divided doses, and monthly evaluations to determine the course of resolution. If, after 6 weeks of therapy no resolution has occurred, we would evaluate the hearing loss in that child with either play audiometry (if the child is old enough) or ABR. If the hearing loss at that time is greater than 30 dB, the child would become a candidate for more aggressive management, which could include either pulse steroids or referral for tympanostomy-tube placement.

Little experience with pulse steroids in young infants has been reported in the treatment of middle ear disease; however, in the treatment of acute asthma, pulse steroids do not appear to be associated with major risks. A consultation with an otolaryngologist and the family will be needed to develop treatment plans. If steroids are chosen, the following dosage regimen has been used: 1 mg/kg per day for 3 or 4 days, 0.5 mg/kg per day for 3 or 4 days, and 0.25 mg/kg per day for 3 or 4 days. Antimicrobial therapy is continued while steroids are initiated. Too little is known, as yet, about pulse steroids to advocate their widespread administration. Careful investigation is necessary to define potential risks and benefits, as well as long-term outcome.

References

1. Teele DW, Klein JO, Rosner B, and Greater Boston Otitis Media Study Group: Epidemiology of otitis media during the first seven years of life in children in Greater Boston: A prospective, cohort study. *J Infect Dis* 1989;160:83.
2. Shurin PA, Pelton SI, Donner A, Klein JO: Persistence of middle ear effusion after acute otitis media in children. *N Engl J Med* 1979;300:1121.
3. Marchant CD, Shurin PA, Turczyk VA, et al: Course and outcome of otitis media in early infancy: A prospective study. *J Pediatr* 1984;104:826.
4. Principi N, Marchisio P, Massironi E, et al: Prophylaxis of recurrent acute otitis media and middle-ear effusion. *Am J Dis Child* 1989;143:1414.
5. Teele DW, Wendall PM, Pelton SI, et al: Prophylaxis in early infancy for infants at risk for otitis media (OM). Abstract #649, presented at the 1990 ICAAC Conference, Atlanta, October 1990.
6. Healy GB: Antimicrobial therapy of chronic otitis media with effusion. *Int J Pediatr Otorhinolaryngol* 1984;8:13.
7. Giebink GS, Batalden PB, Le CT, et al: A controlled trial comparing three treatments for chronic otitis media with effusion. *Pediatr Infect Dis J* 1990;9:33.
8. Berman S, Grose K, Nuss R, et al: Management of chronic middle ear effusion with prednisone combined with trimethoprim-sulfamethoxazole. *Pediatr Infect Dis J* 1990;9:533.
9. Macknin ML, Jones PK: Oral dexamethasone for treatment of persistent middle ear effusion. *Pediatrics* 1985;75:329.

Surgical Management To Decrease Hearing Impairment

Sylvan E. Stool, MD

Point To Recall:
- *Should medical management of otitis media fail, several surgical procedures are available.*

Considerations for Referral:
- *Persistent or recurrent otitis media unresponsive to medical management*
- *Damage to the tympanic membrane or ossicles or other complications of otitis media*

Surgery for prevention or remediation of hearing loss has a long history. In 1801, Sir Astley Cooper published an account in the *Proceedings of the Royal Society* of his procedure for lancing the tympanic membrane and reported the restoration of hearing. He evaluated the patient's auditory acuity using a hunter's watch and noted that if the patient could hear the watch when it was applied to the skull or teeth better than when it was held adjacent to the ear, the operative procedure would be successful. This implies he recognized that he was treating a conductive hearing loss. Subsequently, myringotomy had a number of advocates who soon recognized that the improvement was transient and attempted to keep the opening patent by inserting a stent made of bone or metal or a tube made of rubber.

In the mid-19th century, Adam Politzer, who is considered the father of modern otology, advocated insertion of a grommet fabricated from rubber and acknowledged that the improvement was transient, as the material was extruded. He also advocated inflating the middle ear by applying pressure to the nasopharynx, a method identified as politzeration. Although widely adopted, this procedure was uncomfortable and required frequent office visits.

A method of aerating the middle ear by using a tube was not popular again until the post-World War II era, when the operating microscope became available and new plastic materials were developed. An early proponent of this procedure was Armstrong,[1] whose procedure has subsequently become the most frequently performed minor surgery in children.

There are two major goals for surgery of the ear: to treat or prevent hearing loss and to prevent or correct structural defects. The procedures may involve a tympanic cavity and/or temporal bone or the pharynx.

Tympanocentesis

This procedure involves inserting a needle into the middle ear through the tympanic membrane and is primarily a diagnostic procedure. It is used most frequently to confirm the diagnosis of otitis media, to identify the causative organism if there is a failure of response to therapy, or to recover an unusual organism in an immunocompromised host. The improvement in auditory acuity is usually transient if the ear remains infected.

Myringotomy

This procedure involves an incision in the tympanic membrane and is a therapeutic procedure to evacuate the middle ear cleft. Occasionally, it is used for diagnosis, and it may be used to relieve pain from acute otitis media and provide drainage. Myringotomy may be considered a method of preserving the structure of the tympanic membrane, as it relieves the pressure on a bulging tympanic membrane so that it will not perforate spontaneously and produce an area of necrosis and possibly a permanent perforation.

Myringotomy With Tubes

As mentioned, this is not a new procedure, but one that has been reintroduced. The indications are listed in the Table. A number of clinical studies have been performed in recent years to evaluate the efficacy of the procedure on recurrence of otitis media and treatment of middle ear effusion (MEE).[2,3] Virtually all of these studies agree that the initial hearing improvement is immediate. Thus, if the desired goal of therapy is hearing improvement without delay, this is an effective method of achieving it.[2,3]

Table. Most Frequent Indications for Tympanostomy Tubes in Children.

Treatment failure	Hearing loss
Persistent disease	Prophylaxis
Recurrent infection	Developing structural defect

Sequelae and complications may occur with any procedure. Otorrhea may occur through the tube when the patient has an acute otitis media; this is not considered a complication but a consequence of the patient's disease. The lumen may become obstructed with secretions or blood; this is difficult to prevent when the fluid is thick or there is acute inflammation. The duration of ventilation depends on a number of factors, such as the child's growth and the incidence of infections. Occasionally, a tube will remain for many years. Tympanosclerosis, or thickening of the tympanic membrane, is frequent in ears into which tympanostomy tubes have been inserted; however, it may also occur in ears that have not had surgery. Atrophic scars or retraction pockets may occur at the site of the tube insertion; these are usually of little consequence. Occasionally, a persistent perforation will develop; this may actually be desirable, since it permits middle ear ventilation without a tube. Rarely, a cholesteatoma develops at the site of tube insertion; this is a cyst-like formation.

Granulation tissue can develop around the tube because it acts like a foreign body, and there is bleeding as the tube extrudes. This usually responds to steroid eardrops and antibiotics. The tympanic membrane may grow over the tube or may fill the middle ear, although this is rare and usually does not cause a problem. There has been some concern that tube insertion may cause hearing loss, but cases are extremely rare and may be noted because the child always had a sensorineural hearing loss and did not respond to testing because of the presence of fluid, and it was assumed the fluid was the reason for the loss.

There has been some controversy about the timing of myringotomy with tubes for persistent MEE. Most surgeons agree that MEE may result in the development of retraction pockets in the tympanic membrane, which can lead to cholesteatoma formation.[4] This can destroy the functional tympanic membrane and portions of the temporal bone and, in extreme cases, can even be life-threatening. Myringotomy with tubes and careful follow-up may be effective in halting the progress of this distortion of the tympanic membrane. A much more difficult problem to evaluate is the effect of persistent MEE on the child's subsequent cognitive and emotional development, since it may take years and very carefully controlled studies to demonstrate this effect conclusively. It is only logical to assume that a young child who has difficulty with hearing may also have some emotional or cognitive problem that is not immediately apparent and is due to the fluctuating hearing loss.

Much of the controversy surrounding the importance of ventilating the middle ear may depend on the experience of the physician who is evaluating the child. For instance, an otologist may see patients who have complications and irreversible changes because these are the patients who are referred to him or her, whereas a pediatrician or family practitioner sees the vast majority of patients with MEE, many of whom recover without surgical intervention.

Mastoidectomy

The anatomy of the temporal bone is characterized by an air-cell system that does not contain fluid under normal circumstances. When fluid fills the middle ear and air cells because of infection or eustachian tube obstruction, there will be hearing loss that can be reversed by ventilating the middle ear with a myringotomy or myringotomy and tube. In some instances, there is not good communication between the middle ear and the air-cell system, and fluid persists in the mastoid. Because of the continuing presence of fluid, especially if there is infection, a chronic condition may develop that results in persistent effusion. Surgery is necessary to eradicate the infection from the air-cell system.

Adenoidectomy and Myringotomy

The addition of adenoidectomy and/or tonsillectomy to myringotomy with and without tubes has been investigated. Maw[5] found that adenoidectomy was more effective than no surgery in controlling ear disease. Gates et al,[6] in a study of children 4 to 8 years of age, showed that adenoidectomy and myringotomy with or without tubes was more effective than myringotomy alone with or without tubes. Paradise et al[7] also showed that adenoidectomy in conjunction with tubes in children who had previously had tubes inserted was more effective. These studies are very complex and require careful scrutiny to evaluate their significance.

The decision to do an adenoidectomy is one that may add to the risk or morbidity of the operative procedure and must be weighed against a potential benefit, for, although there appears to be a statistical advantage, the differences in all of the aforementioned studies are not great and the study design was very restrictive.

Tympanoplasty

This procedure is a reconstructive operation to repair damage from previous otitis media. It may require closing a perforation of the tympanic membrane alone or reconstruction of the ossicular chain. In general, it is necessary for the middle ear to be dry, and most surgeons prefer the child to be old enough to cooperate with postoperative care and be out of the age range in which frequent upper respiratory infections are common.

Mastoidectomy and Tympanomastoidectomy

These operations are usually performed when there is persistent otorrhea and are necessary to remove disease from the air-cell system. Hearing may be preserved if the drainage can be controlled and the tympanic membrane can be reconstructed.

The decision for surgical intervention in otitis media is complex. The physician must consider the previous medical therapy and the response to it, the effect of disease on the child and the family, and the age of the patient. The decision can best be made when the family's physician, the family, and the surgeon have all the information available and understand the risk and benefits.

In 1801, in an article in the *Philosophical Transactions of the Royal Society of London,* Sir Astley Cooper summarized his opinion of myringotomy with this statement:

> I have presented several cases in which the joys of hearing have been returned to those who were otherwise deprived of it. Various professional engagements have kept me from devoting sufficient time to this endeavor that I feel it deserves. A knowledge of the ear is by no means prevalent in the profession and still less are its diseases understood. A prejudice has persisted that the tympanic membrane or ear is too delicate of an organ to be operated on or tampered with and thousands have remained deaf throughout their lives because of this. I hope that this paper will dispel this notion and that patients may be restored to the joys of hearing through this simple procedure.

References

1. Armstrong BW: A new treatment for chronic secretory otitis media. *Arch Otolaryngol Head Neck Surg* 1954;59:653.
2. Gebhart DE: Tympanostomy tubes in the otitis media prone child. *Laryngoscope* 1981;91:849.
3. Mandel EM, Rockette HE, Bluestone CD, et al: Myringotomy with and without tympanostomy tubes for chronic otitis media with effusion. *Arch Otolaryngol Head Neck Surg* 1989;115:1217.
4. Bluestone CD, Klein JO: Otitis media, atelectasis, and eustachian tube dysfunction, in Bluestone CD, Stool SE (eds): *Pediatric Otolaryngology.* Philadelphia: WB Saunders Co, 1990, pp 457-464.
5. Maw AR: Chronic otitis media with effusion (glue ear) and adenotonsillectomy: Prospective randomized controlled study. *Br Med J* 1983;287:1586.
6. Gates GA, Avery CA, Prihoda TJ, et al: Effectiveness of adenoidectomy and tympanostomy tubes in the treatment of chronic otitis media with effusion. *N Engl J Med* 1987;317:1444.
7. Paradise JL, Bluestone CD, Rogers KD, et al: Efficacy of adenoidectomy for recurrent otitis media in children previously treated with tympanostomy-tube placement: Results of parallel randomized and nonrandomized trials. *JAMA* 1990;263:2066.

Discussion

Dr Cunningham: I found the comments about trimethoprim-sulfamethoxazole as a prophylactic agent to be of interest, relative to the *Physicians' Desk Reference* statement that this drug is not indicated for long-term prophylaxis.

Dr Klein: Trimethoprim-sulfamethoxazole is likely to be effective for prophylaxis of recurrent episodes of acute otitis media, but the package insert states that the drug is not indicated for prophylaxis or prolonged administration. The physician who chooses to use the drug for this purpose should state in the patient's record the reasons for the choice and should obtain approval from the patient or parent.

Dr Ruben: I have been distressed by the number of children who have been receiving various drugs and who demonstrate allergic reactions or monilial infections.

Dr Pelton: In our studies, *Monilia* was no more common in the children who were given antibiotics than in those who received placebo. We didn't see anyone who had a severely allergic reaction, although one or two children in each group had to stop whichever drug they were on because they had some type of rash that we were concerned was allergic.

Dr Stool: After having treated people for Stevens-Johnson syndrome, I am hesitant to use sulfa, and having seen a child or two die from chickenpox, I am hesitant to use steroids in this age group. I am less hesitant to use amoxicillin.

Dr Pelton: I certainly agree. I am an advocate for amoxicillin as the safest and simplest drug. It should be the drug of first choice.

Dr Hammerschlag: Is there a basis for instituting prolonged multiple courses of antimicrobial therapy?

Dr Pelton: There is no evidence that recurrent courses of antimicrobial agents, if an initial course fails, have anything to do with enhancing the resolution of effusion. These children then become candidates for other approaches. Surgical therapy certainly would be one of those approaches.

Dr Yaffe: The *PDR* contains the product labeling approved by the FDA. If you look in the *PDR* carefully, you see that approximately 80% of the drugs listed are "not for use in infants and children." Physicians should be aware of this labeling.

Dr Pelton, have dose-response studies been done with respect to prednisone? The dose of 1 mg/kg is enormous.

Dr Pelton: The studies have been very narrowly focused on using a pulse of dosing, usually 1 mg/kg for 3 to 5 days, half of that for 3 to 5 days more, and then a quarter of that for another 3 to 5 days. There are no good studies of whether smaller doses or inhaled steroids would be just as effective.

Dr Brookhouser: Let's discuss the problem that none of us wants to see—effusion. You put in a tube and it begins to drain. You have to take the tube back out. The effusion recurs. You're going to have to consider a hearing aid.

Dr Thornton: It would be wonderful if we could convey the concept that hearing aids can be placed for temporary use.

Dr Stool: I think that when you put a tube in, you have to explain to the family that although it does come out of the tympanic membrane, it may not come out of the external canal, and follow-up is necessary. I saw a girl recently who had tubes in for 9 years and had bilateral otorrhea with granulation tissue. Her family had moved frequently and forgot that the tubes had been inserted.

Session VI—
Educational Issues

Educational Implications of Deafness: Language and Literacy

Peter A. de Villiers, PhD

Points To Recall:
- *English-language and literacy development is the primary educational problem for hearing-impaired children.*
- *There is no single answer (such as exposure to sign language) to maximizing literacy skills, since many different language and intellectual factors contribute to fluent reading and writing.*
- *Effective early amplification, facilitation of parent-child communication, and intensive early exposure to the English language in book reading and story sharing enhance acquisition of literacy in the school years.*

Consideration for Referral:
- *Every child with a significant hearing loss should be referred for educational assistance, no matter how young the patient, as soon as the loss is identified.*

Effective English-language skills are essential for the education of deaf students and for the successful integration of deaf individuals into the wider, normally hearing society.[1] However, extensive research over the last 20 to 30 years has documented the limitations of the average hearing-impaired student's English competence over the course of his or her schooling. Although reviews of nationwide achievement testing and demographic data by the Office of Demographic Studies at Gallaudet University[2] reveal a statistically significant improvement in the reading-achievement scores of students in educational programs for the deaf over the last 15 years, the increase is small, and hearing-impaired students typically fall farther and farther behind their normal-hearing peers over the course of their education.

As the top panel of the Figure shows, in the 1990 nationwide norms on the Stanford Achievement Test (SAT), reading-comprehension levels for the average hearing-impaired child increased about two grade equivalents in 8 years of schooling between the ages of 9 and 17 years, reaching approximately the fourth-grade level. The bottom panel provides a contrast of the median mathematics-computation scores for the same population of students. As the Figure makes clear, computational achievement is far less affected by hearing impairment, approaching an eighth-grade level at age 17 years for the average deaf student. On the other hand, as soon as reading is introduced in mathematics word problems, the achievement levels of the children drop to near their reading-comprehension levels. It is apparent from these types of data that the major educational problem for hearing-impaired students is language and literacy acquisition.

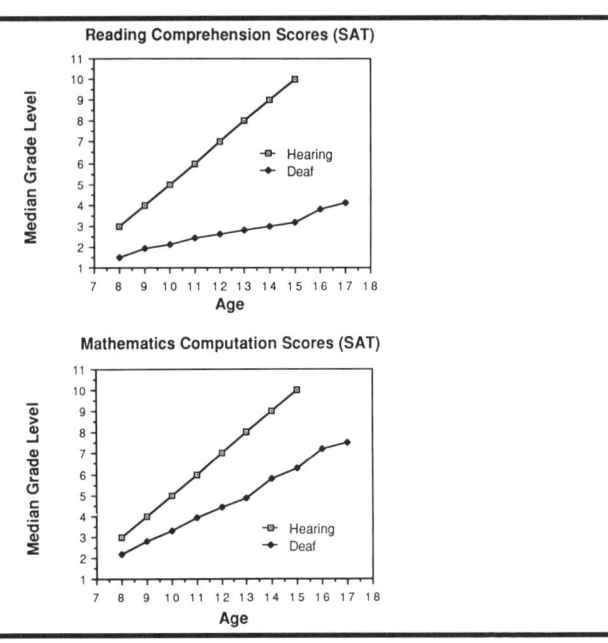

Figure. Median Stanford Achievement Test (SAT) scores in grade levels for the 1990 hearing-impaired population norms. Top panel shows reading-comprehension levels as a function of age (in years) for both normally hearing and hearing-impaired students. Bottom panel shows mathematics-computation scores for the same groups.

English-Language Acquisition, Reading, and Deafness

The normally hearing child and the typical hearing-impaired child are in very different stages of language development when they come to the point of formal schooling and reading instruction. As Table 1 shows, first language acquisition for the normally developing hearing child is rapid and passes through several major milestones in the preschool years, so that when the child reaches formal instruction in reading and writing he or she has a speaking vocabulary of many thousands of words and has mastered in spoken language most of the complex grammar of English. The acquisition of reading is thus primarily learning to map printed English onto an existing knowledge of spoken English.

Although deaf infants begin to babble speech sounds at about the same age as hearing infants do, all the other milestones in the spoken English of deaf children are much delayed. Typically, a few words will be produced by age 24 to 30 months, but 3- and 4-year-olds still have a

Table 1. Milestones in Normal Language Acquisition.

Typical Age	Characteristic Language Development
6-9 months	Repetitive babbling of speech sounds
10-18 months	First recognizable words
15-21 months	Approximately 50 words; onset of rapid vocabulary acquisition
18-30 months	First two- and three-word sentences
30-36 months	Emergence of grammatical function words and markers on verbs and nouns, eg, tenses, plurals, auxiliary verbs
	Range of question forms asked; first "what" and "where," later "why," "when," and "how"
	Joining phrases and sentences with *and*
42-60 months	Beginning acquisition of complex sentence forms—embedded multiverb sentences, adverbial clauses, relative clauses (mastery of these complex forms continues into early school years)
	Productive vocabulary of 5,000-10,000 words

very limited vocabulary of intelligible words, and multiword sentences are rare until the child is about 5 years of age. Verb-tense markers and other grammatical function words (eg, auxiliary verbs *is, are, were, can, does*) and all the complex sentence forms are essentially missing from most deaf children's English language when they reach the early grades of formal schooling, and these aspects of English grammar continue to provide great difficulty for deaf students.[3,4]

Clearly, this varies with degree of hearing loss and effectiveness of early amplification. Provided they do not have other handicapping conditions, children with less-than-severe hearing loss (< approximately 60-dB loss) and consistent early amplification will have some intelligibility problems in their speech. But with appropriate early intervention and preschool language-facilitation programs, they should show only little delay and probably will catch up in their language development by the time they are in regular schooling.

The situation for signing children varies somewhat. For most children who are exposed to signed English forms in the late preschool period and in early schooling, the acquisition of English grammar is similar to that of deaf children in oral programs, with the same delays and areas of difficulty.[5] However, this varies with the completeness of the signed English system they are exposed to, parental signing skill, and the extent of early exposure to the signed language.

In the case of deaf children of deaf parents who communicate with their children in American Sign Language (ASL) from the beginning, the picture is totally different. ASL is acquired as a natural first language by these children, who pass through parallel milestones in grammatical and vocabulary development at about the ages shown in Table 1.[6] But the particulars of the grammatical milestones differ, since ASL is a visual language with grammatical properties quite different from those of spoken English and uniquely suited for the visual mode [see Davis, this publication]. Nevertheless, the percentage of deaf children who acquire ASL as a natural first language is still very small, since deaf children of deaf parents constitute fewer than 10% of all deaf children, and it is extremely rare for a deaf child of hearing parents to be exposed to full ASL early in development. The implications of sign-language acquisition for English-literacy development will be discussed later.

In general, then, the typical deaf child coming to the task of acquiring English-literacy skills is in a very different position from his or her normally hearing peers. By first grade, the normally hearing child has a relatively complete knowledge of the grammar of the language and an extensive vocabulary, but the deaf child is usually lacking much of the required grammatical knowledge and has a severely limited vocabulary. Much of the deaf child's English-language learning therefore comes through printed English, and the task of learning to read is one of *both* cracking the print code *and* learning the language in the first place. The better the child's English-language skills before formal schooling, the easier the task of reading acquisition becomes.

Factors Affecting Reading Achievement: Demographic Studies

Demographic studies reveal several factors relating to the reading achievement of hearing-impaired students.[7] These include

1) Degree of hearing loss. Students with severe hearing impairment (61- to 90-dB loss) had an average reading level of fifth grade at age 17 years; students with profound loss (> 90 dB) averaged mid-third grade at the same age (although this same difference in hearing loss had no effect on mathematics-computation scores).

2) Ethnic background. White students scored significantly higher than black or Hispanic students. This factor involves both socioeconomic and cultural variables, as well as differential access to medical, educational, and other remedial services in these population groups. In the case of many Hispanic students, there is characteristically also the contrast between the use of Spanish language in the home and English language in the school. Very few programs for deaf students are prepared for the educational complexities raised by bilingual spoken-language acquisition as well as the issues of signing and writing English. However, the importance of ethnicity or minority status will continue to grow as minority students make up an increasing percentage of the population of hearing-impaired students.

3) Presence of other handicapping conditions. A significant percentage of students in programs for the deaf are diagnosed with learning disabilities or behavioral problems besides their hearing impairment. The presence of such additional handicapping conditions also adversely affects deaf students' English-literacy development.

Factors Affecting Reading Achievement: Psycholinguistic Studies

Most current theories analyze the global skills of reading and writing into specific psycholinguistic and cognitive components or subskills, although there is some disagreement about the relative weighting that each of the component skills should receive in a complete account of fluent reading. Dominant models of the reading process stress an interaction between *text-based processes*, such as word recognition and print-to-speech/sound decoding, and *inferential processes* involving the use of grammatical, discourse, and experiential knowledge to generate hypotheses or predictions about what the text means and what is coming next as it is read.[8,9]

Different processes may dominate at different points in reading development. Thus, the prereading or early-reading child may be able to "tell" the story of a familiar or highly redundant passage using recognition of few, if any, words and relying almost exclusively on inference and memory of the story events and plot. At a later stage in development, with the beginning of phonics (print-unit to speech/sound-unit correspondence) or whole-word pattern instruction, the child's reading tends to be slow and word by word. However, for fluent reading, both of these processes must be available and must work together. Inferential processes are appropriate when the text content is highly familiar and redundant (we can skim or speed-read such material); but word decoding and sentence-by-sentence grammatical structure must be used when reading text with complex or abstract content.

Factors in Fluent Reading and the Difficulties of Deaf Students

Several language and cognitive processes have been implicated in skilled reading and in the differences between better and poorer readers. These are listed in Table 2. Factors 1, 2, and 3 are related to knowledge of the language and its structure, whereas factors 4 to 7 are related primarily to background knowledge and familiarity with typical reading materials.

In all of these areas, limitations and problems have been reported for deaf students.[10] For example, deaf students understand and use fewer English words across all the different types: nouns, verbs, adjectives, adverbs, and connectives, and the discrepancy between deaf and hearing students becomes even more marked when infrequent, abstract, or multiple-meaning words are tested. Most of our reading vocabulary is acquired by encountering new words in printed text, and there is a close relationship between our vocabulary knowledge and our reading-comprehension skills. Thus, many deaf students are in a vicious circle: Their impoverished vocabularies limit their reading comprehension and poor reading strategies and skills limit their ability to acquire new vocabulary from context.[11]

Table 2. Factors Implicated in Good Reading Development.

1. Vocabulary	Size of vocabulary
	Depth of word knowledge
	Ability to learn words from context
2. Grammar	Understanding of complex sentences and grammatical devices characteristic of written language
3. Phonology	Print-speech/sound decoding
	Awareness of spoken-language structure
4. Discourse/Text Knowledge	Knowledge of the structure of types of text
5. Background/Topic Knowledge	Knowledge of the themes of narratives
	Knowledge of informational topics
6. Inferencing	Ability to infer from what is stated to what is only implied in a passage
7. Metacognition	Monitoring of one's own state of understanding while reading
	Reading-comprehension strategies (knowing where to look for important information)

Hearing impairment has a directly negative effect on the child's access to the speech/sound structure of the language and hence on phonics skills in reading. Yet this is a central component of our decoding of unfamiliar words, and better reading by deaf children is associated with translation of complex sentence structures in written text into a speech-based code rather than a sign-based code.[12]

Similarly, impoverished background knowledge about characteristic topics and themes of children's literature limits the use of inferential processes in reading. Parents typically read much less to their hearing-impaired children than to their normally hearing siblings, and at a later stage impoverished reading skills limit the motivation and the ability to read independently. Furthermore, the past tendency in instructional practice with deaf students to focus on reading isolated sentences and short passages rather than authentic children's stories or longer informational pieces has limited the students' exposure to the characteristic themes and structures of narrative and informational text in English.[13]

The reported difficulties of deaf students with these components of skilled reading can therefore be traced in part to the impact of their hearing loss and in part to the nature of their experience, or lack of it, with the English language, especially in written texts.

Implications for Intervention and Remediation

The preceding sections paint a rather bleak picture of the English-language and literacy achievements of hearing-impaired children, but there are notable successes and positive factors to consider. Significant numbers of even profoundly deaf children achieve English-literacy skills closely comparable with those of their normally hearing peers. High

English-achievement levels close to age level have been reported for groups of children in highly structured, intensive oral programs, in integrated classrooms in mainstream schools, and in some total-communication programs.[14,15]

Some of these high-achieving students have parents who are themselves deaf. In these families, deafness is accepted more readily and the child's social development is considerably enhanced. In many of them, full and natural communication takes place between the parents and child in early development in ASL. But even in deaf families using only oral English, communication between parent and child is maximized, initially with extensive gestural support and later with fluent lip reading. Early exposure to stories and story sharing and to books and book reading is extensive.

Good deaf readers with hearing parents tend to come from families of above-average socioeconomic status and to have parents who are particularly involved in the educational process at home and at school and who have high educational expectations for their children. For these children, whether or not a signed language was used in their educational or home environment, there was early and consistent amplification, as well as early exposure to an intensive English program with a stress on early experience with books and story sharing.

Sign Language and English-Literacy Development

Recently, there has been considerable interest in ASL as a natural language for deaf individuals and as the primary means of social communication within the deaf community. It has even been proposed that ASL serve as the primary medium of instruction in many educational areas and as the means through which English literacy is taught.[16] However, the issue of the best mode of communication to be used in the educational or intervention setting with deaf children remains a contentious one. Indeed, more heat than clarity has been generated in the debate over whether oral English alone, simultaneous spoken and manually encoded English (and if so, which of the several signed English systems), or ASL should provide the primary face-to-face communication system used with the deaf child. Data relevant to these issues are scarce and open to many different interpretations, since the measures of language and educational achievement in existing comparison studies tend to be global and determined by multiple variables. Many of these variables have nothing to do with the modes of communication being compared and cannot be equated across the different populations of students being studied. As a result, the different factions in the debate end up simply disagreeing about the data and arguing largely on ideologic and cultural grounds. Unfortunately, this condition of turmoil in the field of language intervention for the deaf is unlikely to change in the near future.

The fact that this educational area lacks consensus should not dissuade the pediatrician from referring a child for intensive early exposure to language, no matter what system the parents select. Many educational issues, even for normal-hearing children, are controversial, yet there is no question about the importance of early intervention.

What, then, can one conclude about the relationships between signing and English acquisition? First of all, there is no clear evidence that acquisition of a signed language interferes with the acquisition of good English-language and literacy skills, provided the student remains in an environment that also stresses English skills. Second, there is no clear evidence that acquisition of a signed language, either ASL or a manual English form, enhances the acquisition of English reading and writing skills any more than does good oral- and written-English teaching. There is more variation in the success of different educational programs using the same mode of communication than there is between programs using different modes of communication.

Learning ASL in early childhood does provide the child with a natural and complete communication system (an important goal in and of itself), and it may also facilitate the communication of background and content information. But partially because of its many differences from English structure, it does not provide a ready means of acquiring English. In other words, although use of ASL may help with some of the inferential aspects of reading familiar text, it does not facilitate the acquisition of the print-based decoding skills needed for reading complex or unfamiliar passages. Direct instruction in spoken and written English is needed for the latter. Thus, the benefits of signing lie more in facilitating overall communication and social interaction than they do in improving English-literacy skills.

In short, there is no "magic pill" or single solution to overcome the difficulty the deaf child encounters with English-language acquisition. Instead, early, intensive exposure to visual, auditory, and written English in a rich interactional context produces the best outcome in later language skills. Pediatricians and other professionals should encourage parents to maximize early communication with their deaf children by whatever means they can, to become actively involved in an early-intervention program for deaf children that has a strong English program and with which they feel comfortable, and to expose their children to intensive experience with functional English print (eg, signs, labels), books, and book reading.

References

1. *Toward Equality: Education of the Deaf*, A Report to the President and Congress of the United States. Washington: Commission on the Education of the Deaf, 1988.
2. Allen TE: Patterns of academic achievement among hearing-impaired students, in Schildroth AN, Karchmer MA (eds): *Deaf Children in America*. Austin, Tex: PRO-ED Inc, 1986, pp 161-206.
3. Quigley SP, King C: Syntactic performance of hearing-impaired and normal-hearing individuals. *Appl Psycholinguist* 1980;1:329.
4. de Villiers JG, de Villiers PA, Hoban E: The central problem of functional categories in the English syntax of deaf children, in Tager-Flusberg H (ed): *Theoretical Issues in Language Acquisition in Language-Delayed Children*. Hillsdale, NJ: Erlbaum, 1991, pp 83-110.

5. Engen E, Engen T: *The Rhode Island Test of Language Structure*. Austin, Tex: PRO-ED Inc, 1983.
6. Newport E, Meier R: The acquisition of American Sign Language, in Slobin D (ed): *Cross-Linguistic Studies of Language Acquisition*, vol 1: *The Data*. Hillsdale, NJ: Erlbaum, 1985, pp 650-711.
7. Karchmer MA: *1990 Stanford Achievement Test Norms for Hearing-Impaired Students*. Washington: Gallaudet University, Office of Demographic Studies, 1991.
8. Beck I, Carpenter P: Cognitive approaches to understanding reading. *Am Psychol* 1986;41:1098.
9. Rumelhart D: Toward an interactive model of reading, in Dornic S (ed): *Attention and Performance, VI*. New York: Academic Press, 1977, pp 573-603.
10. Quigley SP, Paul P: *Language and Deafness*. Austin, Tex: PRO-ED Inc, 1984.
11. de Villiers PA: English literacy development in deaf children: Directions for research and intervention, in Miller J (ed): *New Directions in the Study of Language Disorders*. Austin, Tex: PRO-ED Inc, 1990, pp 349-378.
12. Lichtenstein E: Deaf working memory processes and English language skills, in Martin D (ed): *International Symposium on Cognition, Education and Deafness*. Washington: Gallaudet University, 1984, pp 331-360.
13. Blackwell P, de Villiers PA, Hoffmeister R: *English Literacy Acquisition in Deaf Children*, Grant report to the National Institute on Disability and Rehabilitation Research, 1991.
14. Geers AE, Moog JS: *Factors Predictive of the Development of Reading and Writing Skills in the Congenitally Deaf: Report on the Oral Sample*. NIH-NINCDS Report, 1987.
15. Moores D: *Factors Predictive of Literacy in Deaf Adolescents*. NIH-NINCDS Report, 1987.
16. Johnston J, Liddell S, Erting C: *Unlocking the Curriculum: Principles for Achieving Access in Deaf Education*, Gallaudet Research Institute Working Paper 89-3. Washington: Gallaudet University, 1989.

Evaluation, and Then What? What Pediatricians Should Know About Hearing Loss in Young Children

Dennis Gjerdingen, MS

Points To Recall:
- *All children, no matter how young, can be tested.*
- *Parents must understand a hearing loss in their child.*
- *Childhood deafness is an educational, more than a medical, challenge.*

Consideration for Referral:
- *Refer to trained, licensed audiologists or otologists who are experienced with hearing-impaired children whenever a hearing loss is suspected.*

Parents usually share their first suspicions about their child's hearing loss with their pediatrician. The pediatrician is in a position to confirm the parents' worst fear—that the child is deaf. Although a diagnosis of childhood deafness is devastating to a family,[1] steps can be taken to reduce the effects of deafness on development. I speak as the parent of a deaf son and as a professional who works with parents. Specifically, I suggest linking families to professionals who are experienced in working with young deaf children.

The Clarke School for the Deaf/Center for Oral Education has more than a century of experience with deaf children and provides the background for this topic. Clarke is internationally known as a school, as a center for research and professional preparation, and, more recently, as a multifaceted center developed around the philosophy of preparing hearing-impaired individuals to function independently in our society. Annually, the audiologists see more than 300 children under the age of 3 years, the early-intervention center deals with more than 100 families, and the mainstream center provides technical assistance to more than 100 hearing-impaired children in classes with hearing children. In addition, dozens of children are evaluated in the comprehensive educational evaluation program and in the school-admissions process.

This extensive experience with deaf children has led us to create three principles: 1) Hearing loss in infants and young children can be identified early. 2) Parents must understand their child's hearing loss and the implications for development. 3) Childhood deafness is a long-term educational issue.

Too often, parents state that a pediatrician dismissed their early suspicions of the child's poor response to sound with a statement such as "Don't worry about that; different children react differently at different ages. Your child will respond when he wants to. Just give him time." Parents also comment that "An article said that a child with an older sibling will not talk as much because the older sibling will talk for her"; or "I was told that boys are always slower to talk than girls because boys are more active."

Speech and language development should be observed and monitored by *all* professionals involved in the care of infants and toddlers. We continue to see children over the age of 2 years who do not speak or who speak in single words, understood only by familiar adults. Even mild, temporary hearing losses such as those resulting from otitis media should be treated and monitored. A child with a history of chronic otitis media is at risk for speech and language delays, as well as for academic and behavioral problems in the classroom. The severity of secondary consequences is directly related to the severity and frequency of the conductive loss.

We have developed a profile of children with chronic otitis media [unpublished]. These children are not interested in sound and they have difficulty concentrating on an activity if it requires listening. Sound is not meaningful to them. They do not trust their ears to provide them with consistent information about the environment, so they do not pay attention to sound. Parents of children with chronic middle ear problems describe them as "bouncing off the walls," being uncooperative, or having other disruptive behaviors. It appears that these children are attempting to control their environment through inappropriate behavior since they cannot control it with language. With medical/surgical intervention and aggressive management, the prognosis for eliminating secondary effects is good.

The potential impact of a unilateral hearing loss is also misunderstood and should not be underestimated. An outdated school of thought is that as long as one ear has normal hearing, speech and language will develop normally and academic difficulties will be minimized. However, recent research[2] suggests that children with a unilateral loss are at risk for academic difficulties.

A child is never too young for a hearing test. The test for middle ear dysfunction, tympanometry, is objective, quick, and reliable. Testing methods for diagnosing sensorineural impairment are more complicated and vary according to the child's age and abilities. Behavioral evaluations do not rule out a mild degree of hearing loss in the very young infant; however, such testing can rule out or identify a hearing loss that will significantly affect the development of speech and language. Auditory brain-stem response (ABR) testing, an objective electrophysiologic test, is widely available and can be used to confirm behavioral results. The sooner a hearing impairment is identified, the sooner the habilitative procedures can begin.

Even if the initial evaluation rules out a significant hearing loss, routine monitoring every few months may be recommended, especially if the child is at risk for hearing loss [see **Appendix A**]. Monitoring permits the audiologist to observe the development of auditory behavior and to identify a progressive loss. For example, a child who was identified as having a severe hearing loss at age 3½ months was found to have progressed to a profound loss in less than 2 months. If this child had been evaluated only once in 6 to 12 months, he would have spent his first 6 months using a hearing aid that was not appropriate for his loss. Although such a progressive hearing loss may not be common, it is every audiologist's ethical responsibility to monitor hearing very closely until the loss is stabilized.

Audiologists use standardized norms that correlate auditory development with behavioral response. The behavioral response to sound changes as the infant matures and gains experience with sound. It is important to note that these norms are reported in terms of "developmental age," not chronologic age. Developmental age is adjusted for premature delivery; for example, it is expected that an 8-week-old infant born 6 weeks prematurely will have auditory behavior commensurate with that of a 2-week-old child. Developmental age adjustment must also be applied to children who are developmentally delayed. At Clarke, two professionals test all children; one presents the stimuli while the other controls the child's attention. This procedure increases the validity of the observations by increasing the number of observers. It also eliminates the parent as a biased observer. Two experienced observers also reduce the length of the test time, which is critical in view of a young child's limited attention span.

Results from behavioral testing of very young children should be corroborated with ABR testing. For example, an 18-month-old child was evaluated who did not respond to auditory stimuli at the output limit of the audiometer on three separate occasions. Yet the ABR was normal for both ears, strongly suggesting that this was a case of a central hearing loss. Without supplemental ABR testing, however, the child would have been inappropriately fitted with powerful hearing aids.

A child is never too young to use amplification. Audiologists may have different opinions on the appropriate form of amplification for an infant (eg, ear-level hearing aids versus body aids versus FM systems), but they agree that a child is never too young to be fitted with an amplification device.

Pediatricians often feel limited in their ability to advise parents in cases of suspected severe-to-profound hearing impairments. Our advice is to listen carefully to the parents' concerns. If there is reasonable doubt about the functioning of the auditory system, refer the child for testing immediately. It is important to establish a relationship with a test center staffed with qualified and licensed audiologists who also have experience with young deaf children. In the long run, parents will be better served by the most qualified audiologist, even if he or she is not the one closest to home. Conscientious audiology-clinic personnel know the importance of early detection and will make adjustments in a full schedule to see a young child referred by a physician. For example, although we generally have a 6-week waiting list for an appointment in our clinic, a referring pediatrician can expect that we will shift schedules so that we see a child within 2 days.

The discussion so far has dealt with children. The second principle focuses on parents. Parents must have a working knowledge of hearing loss. Parents usually demonstrate a strong emotional reaction when their child's hearing loss is confirmed. Generally, they have suspected some degree of hearing loss and may appear quite rational when it is confirmed. However, experience has shown that trying to give them a great deal of technical information in a short period is not effective. The information is best conveyed over a longer period in different sessions, supplemented with visual aids and analogies, and restated in writing. Rarely do parents take in all the information provided by an audiogram, since familiarity with the symbols and technical terminology is necessary.

To provide an effective environment for their children, parents must come to understand the nature, severity, and implications of the loss on a child's development. Breaking the information down into simple steps and easy-to-understand language, over a period of time, helps the parents comprehend the implications for the future. Since parents may direct questions about interpreting an audiogram to pediatricians, we suggest Boothroyd[3] as a helpful guide. However, the sooner the parents are under the care of a certified, experienced educational audiologist or teacher of the deaf, the sooner the family will begin to work toward long-term solutions.

Our third principle, that childhood deafness is an educational issue more than a medical one, is without a doubt the most difficult principle for the medical community to comprehend. Physicians are trained to prevent, correct, and cure medical problems. Currently, there is no cure for deafness. Even surgical procedures such as cochlear implantation are not a cure for hearing loss. The success of the implant in children relies heavily on the program of rehabilitation and education that follows the surgery. In general, an implant gives a child who is totally deaf access to acoustic information equivalent to that of a profoundly deaf child. Furthermore, the public is aware that there is disagreement within the educational community about the oral or manual management of deaf children. Physicians are reluctant to refer parents into what appears to be confusion. However, the reality is that a sensorineural loss is permanent, and the sooner parents can become active in choosing an appropriate educational path, the better the prognosis for the child.

After 25 years in education of the deaf, as a parent, as a professional, and as a national representative on deaf-education issues, I can safely say that the controversy over how a deaf child is best educated has no visible end. It is important for the medical community to know that there is no single way to educate all deaf children, only different choices. It is important to preserve those alternatives and to help parents make informed choices about what might be best for each family with its unique set of circumstances. Therefore, the best advice for pediatricians is to acquaint themselves with the available options and with a representative professional so that they can refer parents to different approaches, from which the parents can educate themselves and make their own decisions.

Auditory/Oral Education

I have been asked to address some specific questions about auditory/oral education from my experience. Decisions about the appropriateness of any educational program should stem from a comprehensive evaluation. In addition to defining the child's hearing ability, this evaluation also describes the child's ability to learn along with providing important information about what might be impeding that learning. It should also include an assessment of the child's academic, speech, and language progress.

Following such an evaluation, an individualized educational plan should be written that reflects the child's needs. The Commission on the Education of the Deaf drafted important considerations that need to be observed when making decisions about educational placements for deaf students; parents are a vital component in such decisions.[4]

There are no simple criteria to identify a child who might do better in an auditory/oral setting than in a setting where signing is emphasized. In general, the more hearing present, the more intelligible the speech.[5]

However, English-language acquisition, an area in which we have done much recent research, does not correlate highly with hearing ability or speech intelligibility. It is the lack of English-language competence, much more than poor speech, that becomes the disabling factor of deafness. To a great extent, poor English-language ability is responsible for the low reading level (at or below the fourth-grade level[6]) of deaf youngsters when they graduate from high school.

Of more than 300 students who completed our program and went on to high school in the last decade, only 5 did not complete their program. Over 80% of our students have gone on to postsecondary education at more than 200 different colleges, universities, and other programs. Some of our alumni have doctorates, master's, and other degrees, and their occupations range from architect and scientist through a wide scope of careers.[7]

Since 1867, the Clarke philosophy has been that individuals who are deaf can be prepared to live independent and productive lives in the mainstream of society. Clarke was the first school to place students who were deaf in the mainstream, over 100 years ago. Today, mainstreaming has become the law of the land. Unfortunately, many public schools, their deaf students, and those students' families have not been adequately prepared to make mainstreaming a successful educational experience. In addition, most regular schools are not adequately supported with technical assistance for their deaf students. Mainstream education can and does work,[8] with much guidance and support to the students, parents, and schools. It is not a simple educational placement, however, and it is not for all deaf children.

Conclusion

Whenever a pediatrician suspects a hearing loss in an infant or a child, the greatest service he or she can provide for the family is an appropriate referral to a certified audiologist who is experienced in working with deaf children in an educational setting and who works in conjunction with educators experienced with children who are deaf.

~

To learn more about mainstream education for deaf students, pediatricians and/or families can contact The Mainstream Center, Clarke School for the Deaf/Center for Oral Education, in Northampton, Massachusetts [see **Appendix B**] or The Alexander Graham Bell Association for the Deaf, 3417 Volta Place NW, Washington, DC 20007 (202/337-5220).

Recommended Readings
    Davis H, Silverman SR: *Hearing and Deafness*, ed 4. New York: Holt Rinehart & Winston, 1978.
    Gatty J: The oral approach: A professional point of view, in Schwartz S (ed): *Choices in Deafness, a Parent's Guide*. Kensington, Md: Woodbine House, 1987, pp 57-64.

Manning FD: Supportive mainstreaming from a residential school, in Ross M (ed): *Hearing-Impaired Children in the Mainstream.* Parkton, Md: York Press Inc, 1991, pp 213-228.

References
1. Luterman D: *Counseling the Communicatively Disordered and Their Families.* Boston: Little Brown & Co, 1984.
2. Oyler R, Oyler A, Matkin N: Unilateral hearing loss: Demographics and educational impact. *Lang Speech Hear Serv Schools* 1988;19:201.
3. Boothroyd A: *Hearing Impairments in Young Children.* Englewood Cliffs, NJ: Prentice-Hall Inc, 1982, pp 221-225.
4. *Toward Equality: Education of the Deaf,* A Report to the President and Congress of the United States. Washington: Commission on the Education of the Deaf, 1988.
5. Boothroyd A: Residual hearing and the problems of carry-over in the speech of the deaf. *ASHA Rep* 1985;15:8.
6. Allen T: *Understanding the Scores: Hearing-Impaired Students and the Stanford Achievement Test,* ed 7. Washington: Gallaudet Research Institute Center for Assessment and Demographic Studies, 1986.
7. Blish S: *A Survey of the Educational and Vocational Experiences of the Alumni of the Clarke School for the Deaf.* Northampton, Mass: Clarke School for the Deaf, 1981.
8. Gjerdingen D, Manning FD: Adolescents with profound hearing impairments in mainstream education: The Clarke model in selected issues in adolescence and deafness. *Volta Rev* 1991;93:139.

Signing and Total Communication
Julia M. Davis, PhD

Points To Recall:
- Sign language is one of several habilitative strategies that should be considered for deaf children.
- The choice of educational method and placement for a given child must be based on assessment of the child's learning style.

Consideration for Referral:
- Hearing loss in any child whose parents wish to know all educational options available

Two major trends have occurred in the education of hearing-impaired children during the last 25 years. The first of these is the widespread acceptance of total communication (TC) as a tool for educating and communicating with deaf children. The second is the placement of hearing-impaired children in regular classrooms for most of their academic instruction; this situation is called *mainstreaming.* The two trends are not entirely compatible.

TC refers to an educational philosophy in which every possible sensory avenue is used to transmit information to deaf children and to facilitate their expression of language. TC includes the use of amplified sound to stimulate the damaged auditory system; finger spelling, lip reading, gestures, and formal signs that can be received through the visual system; and touch, vibrations, and movement to allow information to be processed through the tactile and proprioceptive systems. The child receives input through all available sensory systems, allowing those that are intact to compensate for the damaged auditory system. The child is also encouraged to use speech, sign, finger spelling, and gestures to express language. This approach is meant to be eclectic, and over time a child may reject some components in favor of others, thus maximizing individual strengths and communicative styles. This philosophy recognizes the uniqueness of children's learning styles and communicative needs; it does not presume that one style is superior to any other.

One essential cornerstone of TC is sign language. Unfortunately, for some educators and observers, it has become the only component associated with TC, setting the stage for intense controversy in the context of what would appear to be a sound and logical approach toward a difficult educational task.

TC is often compared to oral education. In actual practice, elements of each are contained in the other approach. TC includes lip reading, auditory input, and speech training. Oral programs include gestures for ease of communication. Both types of programs have much to offer hearing-impaired children if procedures are matched to children's needs. A child who has very little hearing and only in the low frequencies is unlikely to learn as rapidly through auditory input as through the visual system. Conversely, a child with significant residual hearing at all frequencies should be able to make good use of auditory input and may not need to rely on visual information for maximum performance. A careful evaluation of the individual child's abilities is essential to educational planning.

Mainstreaming refers to an educational philosophy first represented in Public Law 94-142, the Education for All Handicapped Children Act. In essence, this law requires that handicapped children be educated in the "least restrictive environment" possible. The intent of the law is to prevent isolation of handicapped children by placing them in regular classrooms whenever possible. The law has had little effect on hard-of-hearing children, who were almost always mainstreamed anyhow, but it has had a significant effect on many children with profound hearing impairment. Without adequate support services, including on-site interpreters, these children cannot participate effectively in a classroom in which the teacher is not trained to present information to children who cannot hear and which does not have adequate acoustics. When classmates have no understanding of the effects of hearing loss on a child's ability to communicate, the social effect of mainstreaming can be quite negative. The overall result has often been a more, rather than a less, restrictive environment for deaf children, many of whom report a deep sense of frustration and isolation.

Use of Sign Language

One of the first factors to consider when choosing educational options for deaf children is whether or not to include sign language. This is the most controversial aspect of the management of hearing loss by parents and professionals. By the early 1900s, most schools for the deaf offered oral education exclusively during the first 5 to 7 years of school, introducing sign language only when oral instruction failed to result in adequate educational achievement. Proponents of the use of sign language were accused of interfering with the development of the lip-reading and speech skills necessary for deaf children to function in a hearing world. In turn, oral educators were accused of wasting the early period of children's lives, known to be important for language development. It is far easier for the average deaf child to learn a sign for a given object, act, or state than to learn a word; deaf children as young as 12 or 13 months have learned to use a sign that represents a relevant object (eg, candy) after a single exposure to it. Through lip reading and audition, a thousand repetitions might be necessary to learn the same word, and then the child might not be able to express it orally.

Not until the concept of TC was introduced in the 1960s did sign language become a widely accepted component of preschool education. By 1975, the majority of educational programs had incorporated sign language into their procedures. Even so, the topic is still controversial and its future use is likely to be as variable as in the past. Why so much emotion about this particular legal use of the hands?

The controversy centers around a single question: What is the best way to teach deaf children to communicate well enough to be educated, productive citizens? For children in this country, mastery of the English language is the standard. The fact that there can be no single teaching strategy that is best for all hearing-impaired children has not diminished the heat of the arguments presented by those who favor and those who oppose the use of sign language. For at least 100 years, the arguments on either side were based almost entirely on emotion and rhetoric, rather than on empiric evidence regarding the degree to which manual communication was either successful or detrimental to deaf children. By the early 1960s, there was considerable discontent among educators, parents, deaf adults, and professional persons who worked with deaf individuals. The educational achievement of deaf children was very low; the average reading achievement after 10 to 12 years of special education was at the fourth-grade level, and fully 30% of deaf teenagers were functionally illiterate.[1-3] Oral education was blamed by many for the failure of the average deaf child to achieve academically.

Between 1960 and 1980, several investigators reported studies of the effects of the early use of sign language on the educational, social, and linguistic development of deaf children.[1,2,4-9] Performance by the deaf children of deaf parents was compared to that of deaf children of hearing parents. In study after study, the children of deaf parents who had been exposed to sign language from birth showed significantly higher academic achievement, better social adjustment, and lip-reading and speaking skills that were equal to or better than those of deaf children who had not been exposed to manual communication early in life. Stevenson[1] reported that 38% of a manually trained group he studied attended college, whereas only 9% of an orally trained group did so.

These data must be interpreted cautiously. The studies were conducted with children who were not identified as hearing-impaired in infancy and who, therefore, did not receive special educational services early in life. Furthermore, there have been significant improvements in amplification devices and their selection procedures in recent years. Today's deaf children might respond differently, although the data collected periodically by the Gallaudet College Office of Demographic Studies reveal only minor improvements in average academic achievement since these studies were reported.

The studies reported here reflect the enormous importance of establishing a language base early in any child's life. Hearing children have learned the essential components of their native language by the age of 3 or 4 years. Many deaf children are not even identified until they are between 1 and 3 years of age; by then, their development of the English language is already seriously delayed. Obviously, the more language these children can learn quickly, the better their chances of reducing the impact of deafness on eventual achievement. We must remember, however, that oral language is learned most naturally and speech is monitored most effectively through the auditory system. If the goal is proficiency in oral language—and it usually is—every possible effort must be made to stimulate children auditorily, whether sign language is used or not.

It is essential that the optimal learning style of each child be identified as early as possible. For this reason, early selection of amplification, close monitoring, and diagnostic teaching by an audiologist, speech-language pathologist, and/or educator of the deaf is essential to a child's future psycholinguistic performance. When there is doubt about the efficiency of the auditory system for learning language, both auditory stimulation and manual communication should probably be provided.[9] This is the essence of the TC approach as it was originally proposed. The data reported by Moores et al[10] show clearly that the children who perform best on a variety of language measures are those who have the most residual hearing and who are enrolled in TC programs that emphasize auditory stimulation in addition to sign language.

At the same time, it is now clear that deaf children exposed to sign language as infants are able to master considerable vocabulary and learn the basic rules of grammar at about the same time and in the same sequence as hearing children. It is not unusual for children of deaf parents to babble in sign and to produce common signs as early as 6 to

8 months of age. The neuromotor coordination required to produce an understandable sign is less than that required to produce words, so deaf children who are exposed to sign language from birth often use their first "words," that is, signs, several months earlier than their hearing peers use words.

Most deaf infants, however, are born to hearing parents who have had no experience with deafness or with sign language. They are not yet aware of the full impact that deafness may have on learning, communication, and psychosocial development. Their immediate focus is on speech: the child's ability to understand what is said and to produce messages by speaking. Sign language may not be introduced early because it is as alien to these parents as sound is to their children. Studies[11] show that delayed introduction of language through signs does not hamper the development of vocabulary and basic word order. However, a delay usually results in reduced ability to use the morphology of the English language correctly.[11] Sign language must not be presented as the panacea for a deaf child's problems, because it never can be. Although many studies show that deaf children who learn sign in infancy perform better than other deaf children in a number of areas, including the use of the English language, their performance is still far below that of hearing children.

To Sign or Not To Sign?

Parents expect professionals to give them advice about major decisions that will affect both the hearing-impaired child and the rest of the family. Some parents prefer that professionals make the major decisions for them. This is not a good idea, and we should resist it strongly. Nevertheless, professionals must serve as objective information providers and advisors. On the issue of whether or not to introduce sign language to a given child, three points should be considered.

Age at Identification and Intervention

The longer the hearing loss is undetected and untreated, the greater the language deficit. Children who are not identified before the age of 3 years may require multisensory stimulation to encourage rapid language growth. Under these circumstances, it may be important to introduce sign language along with auditory stimulation early in the child's habilitation. If the child demonstrates the ability to learn quickly through the auditory system, manual communication can be phased out as dependence on it decreases. If the child requires more visual input in order to learn, it will not have been withheld at a critical period in the child's life.

Availability of Educational Options

The educational philosophy and procedures of local programs for hearing-impaired children may determine the advice given to parents. Unless more than one option is available, parents may be frustrated and confused by a recommendation for educational programming that does not exist locally. When there is a severe mismatch between what is available and the child's needs, parents must be encouraged to consider educational placement outside the local community, either at a residential school for the deaf or on a day basis in a neighboring community. Information about educational programs across the country can be found each year in the May-June issue of *American Annals of the Deaf*.

Parental Preference

In the final analysis, the decision about whether or not to use sign language with a given child rests with the parents. Once they have been given information about the child's hearing loss and the different educational approaches that may be appropriate, the parents should be encouraged to discuss their feelings about the options available. Pediatric audiologists are especially well prepared to help parents explore their reactions to the diagnosis of deafness and their role in the child's habilitation. Every effort should be made to refer children to these specialists as soon as hearing impairment is suspected.

References

1. Stevenson E: A study of the educational achievement of deaf children of deaf parents. *Calif News* 1964;80:143.
2. Denton D: A study in the educational achievement of deaf children, in *Report of the Proceedings of the 42nd Meeting of the Convention of American Instructors of the Deaf*. Washington: US Government Printing Office, 1966, pp 428-433.
3. McClure W: Current problems and trends in the education of the deaf. *Deaf Am* 1966;18:223.
4. Stuckless E, Birch J: The influence of early manual communication on the linguistic development of deaf children. *Am Ann Deaf* 1966;111:452.
5. Meadow K: Early manual communication in relation to the deaf child's intellectual, social, and communicative functioning. *Am Ann Deaf* 1968;113:29.
6. Vernon M, Koh S: Effects of oral preschool compared to early manual communication in deaf children. *Am Ann Deaf* 1971;116:569.
7. Balow I, Brill R: An evaluation of reading and academic levels of sixteen graduating classes of the California School for the Deaf. *Volta Rev* 1975;77:255.
8. Brasel K, Quigley S: The influence of certain language and communication environments in early childhood on the development of language in deaf individuals. *J Speech Hear Res* 1977;20:95.
9. Moores D: *Educating the Deaf*. Boston: Houghton Mifflin Co, 1978, p 61.
10. Moores D, Weiss K, Goodwin M: Early education programs for hearing impaired children: Major findings. *Am Ann Deaf* 1978;123:925.
11. Meier RP: Language acquisition by deaf children. *Am Sci* 1991;79:60.

Discussion

Ms Tucker: Dr de Villiers, a controversy centers around the better way to educate deaf children, to sign or to speak. I prefer to think that the controversy really is, What goals do you want these deaf children to attain? Do you want them to be part of the mainstream of society, in which case they will have to communicate orally, or do you want them to be part of a deaf subculture?

Dr de Villiers: There is no evidence that the acquisition of a sign language interferes with the acquisition of English-language skills, whether they are spoken or written. The data depend crucially on the kind of program the students are in. If they are in a program that neglects training in speech skills, they will not develop good speech skills. If I had a personal preference, it would be for deaf children to have an opportunity to learn sign language, should they and their parents desire it, but for the children also to have full exposure to English.

Dr Brookhouser: The physician must be an advocate—not an advocate for any system, but an advocate for the child. Parents are so frustrated. They are getting conflicting opinions about what ought to be done. It is very important that physicians not take sides on these issues, but keep constantly returning the burden of decision to the parents.

Dr Stool: Many parents and many physicians do not understand that the child who is deaf is vulnerable to middle ear disease. The child already does not hear, to provide a clinical clue; the child may not speak well, to complain of pain. So the otitis media goes untreated.

It is also important for physicians to realize that educators want to save money. It costs a lot less to mainstream a child to a local school than for the school system to pay to send the child to a school for the deaf. Many children do very well with mainstreaming, but if a child does not, somewhere along the line society will have a higher price to pay.

Dr Eavey: How would a parent seek out a school or advice from educators about the best educational milieu for their child?

Dr Davis: The recently revised book *Our Forgotten Children: Hard of Hearing Pupils in the Schools** [Davis J (ed); US Dept of Education, 1990] contains a chapter by a parent who has challenged a school system and won better services for his child and a chapter by an official in a school system who tells parents how to work through the bureaucracy to get services that are required for their children.

Mr Gjerdingen: The decision about education really requires an intensive evaluation. You must be able to look at an individual child and his or her needs. There are auditory needs, but those are not the most important ones. You must look at the psychologic needs and at the

---

*Available for a nominal cost from Self Help for Hard of Hearing People, 7800 Wisconsin Ave, Bethesda, MD 20814

child's learning capabilities. The one recommendation I really agree with is to honor parent preference. If parents aren't happy with what they are doing with their own child, nothing else is going to matter. That information is not as hard to develop as people think it is. It's just that there aren't very many places where all the specialists who need to sit on an evaluation team are available at the same time.

Dr Hart: The child's audiologist or otolaryngologist and primary-care physician should meet the family together, no matter how difficult that might be to arrange.

Ms Tucker: There is an assumption that the more profoundly deaf a child is, the less likely it is that speech will come. I don't believe that's true. That is one factor, but only one of many different factors. We are sitting here with two profoundly deaf people who speak very well.

Session VII—
Personal Experience

Reflections of a Hearing-Impaired Otologist
Paul E. Hammerschlag, MD

Points To Recall:
- *Hearing loss is invisible; the physician should consider audiologic tests when there is a genetic history, parental concern, known high-risk factors, only one hearing ear, or meningitis.*
- *Hearing loss is insidious and may lead to language delay.*
- *An early window of opportunity exists for aural rehabilitation.*
- *Aural rehabilitation should begin in infancy or as soon as possible after a diagnosis of significant hearing impairment is made.*

I confess that I am ambivalent about reflecting at this forum, where most of us were invited for our ability to contribute on an objective scientific basis. Subjective reflections certainly are not necessarily comparable to insights derived from scientific analysis.

I have been asked to suggest some aspects of my personal experience that will reinforce and focus the scientific points presented at this conference. I hope that the sharing of my past will imbue the primary-care physician with a sense of urgency and direction in managing the invisible problem of childhood hearing loss. While I speak primarily as an otologist with some experience with these children, I should like to share with you the need to impart a positive sense of direction and purpose to the distraught parents of children with newly identified hearing loss. Such empiric direction is part of the art of medicine, which all clinicians variably practice.

That I am mainstreamed as an oral communicator is not to suggest that this method is intrinsically superior to sign or total communication. Since oral communication was the only option made available to me, alternative methods of communication were precluded. Realistically, oral communication using the language of our mainstream society is the only direct means of verbal communication without an interpreter.

My story begins in the late 1940s, when reliable and accurate pediatric audiology was not available. Because of delayed speech development, at the age of 2½ years I was placed in a speech-therapy program with a Viennese speech therapist whose claim to fame was that he allegedly had trained a dog to talk. I recall this not to ridicule the gentleman but to emphasize how desperately illogical and confused my parents were initially.

During this period, the possibility of a hearing loss was also raised, and amplification with a hearing aid was recommended. Because a hearing loss could not be satisfactorily confirmed to my parents, they were reluctant to proceed with such amplification. At that time, my paternal grandfather was the only family member with a severe hearing loss that required a hearing aid. My father, a physician, was certainly bewildered by the myriad opinions and conflicting expert advice. Some people suggested hearing aids for an unconfirmed hearing loss; some suggested that there was no evidence for hearing loss; others suggested radiation therapy to the nasopharynx for eustachian tube dysfunction; and others raised the question of psychologic impairment.

When I was 4 years old, a hearing loss was identified by what was then thought to be a valid method: psychogalvanic skin testing, which was performed at the Johns Hopkins Hospital. This test was based on identification of perspiration from the skin induced by auditory stimuli associated with electric shocks after a period of conditioning. Several years later, the accuracy of this method was demonstrated to be inconsistent. Nevertheless, my parents felt by that time that there was sufficient confirmation of a hearing loss to explain my delayed language and lack of speech. At the age of $4\frac{1}{2}$ years, I was finally fitted with a hearing aid. It was a bulky body aid with a "button" in one ear.

In contrast to the preceding, accurate auditory assessment certainly can be obtained today in the first several months of life with skilled pediatric audiology. Precise auditory evaluation may be delayed in infants with mental retardation or psychomotor deficits. Auditory brain-stem testing, even with its limitations, can be a powerful diagnostic tool for early auditory evaluation.

Contemporary pediatricians certainly would be more suspicious of a hearing loss and would more aggressively establish a diagnosis earlier, especially in a family with paternal hearing loss. Ultimately, genetic pedigree analysis documented that my hearing loss was a dominant hereditary type with variable expression and progression with age. With the active role of genetics and dysmorphology units in most modern pediatric training programs, there is a heightened awareness of hereditary aspects of disease, which should enhance earlier identification of deafness associated with a family history or with certain syndromes. More complete care can be attained with referral for genetic counseling, enrollment in a genetic registry, and, in some facilities, possible molecular genetic analysis.

Returning to my history, intensive aural rehabilitation was initiated in association with aural amplification with a hearing aid. This therapy consisted of hour-long individualized sessions four or five times a week in which I was taught to speak primarily by first learning to read. Auditory information and the visually perceived printed word were synergistically taught to me so that I could acquire speech and language. I had the distinct and fortunate advantage to benefit from intensive individualized therapy, in contrast to those who were rehabilitated in classes, which I also attended. With all things being equal, I believe that those of us who were fortunate to have successful intensive individual therapy developed language and communication skills superior to those of people who received therapy in groups or classes. The building blocks of language are best taught on a one-to-one basis. After language and communication skills are acquired, the hearing-impaired child should be better able to participate in preschool and elementary-school curricula.

I believe that had auditory rehabilitation commenced in my infancy, I would now have a better-developed auditory neural substrate, which would enable me to hear better with my residual hearing. With a 4-year delay in my developing language, followed by intensive efforts in visual-oral communication, my auditory skills were never fully developed, resulting in what I call mild "auditory dyslexia," for lack of a better term. To this day, I have to think about and interpret or process what I hear, as opposed to just responding immediately. Frequently, I repeat what has been said, either to confirm that I have heard correctly or to acquire extra time to process this material. I feel that this circuitous method of processing auditory information is due to incomplete development of residual auditory skills secondary to a more-favored dependency on visual skills, ie, lip reading.

Reduced auditory skills may also be due to a dependency on the printed word, particularly if reading is the major source of language acquisition and education. The printed word was and is my language: When I hear a word, the printed word frequently comes to mind simultaneously, which may also delay my processing of simultaneously rendered aural and visual information, especially in a classroom setting. On the other hand, without the printed word from reading, I probably would not have had any mainstream oral language.

Today, a significantly greater proportion of children with severe to profound hearing loss have language skills sufficient to allow them to be successfully mainstreamed. This is most likely due to early initiation of auditory rehabilitation. These children are initially fitted with FM units that give clearer auditory input via transmission of speech from a wireless microphone worn by a speaker; this reduces ambient noise and improves the signal-to-noise ratio. This uncontaminated speech renders auditory information superior to that provided by conventional hearing aids, for more effective input during the language-formation years (0 to 5-7 years).

In terms of speech therapy and auditory input with these FM units in and out of the home, a linguistic foundation is established that later enables children to be mainstreamed with hearing aids. In my youth and over the years, the majority of these children with severe to profound hearing loss failed to develop the language and communication skills that would have allowed them to be successfully mainstreamed. Therefore, I am amazed at how well some of these children are doing with the FM unit in terms of rehabilitation programs. It seems that these earliest years represent a crucial window of time during which one can optimally acquire language. If it is not attained by the age of 5 or 7 years, these children will continue to fall behind their peers, who will be learning other skills based on their established communicative abilities.

For myself and for those children who are successfully mainstreamed today, active, sustained parental participation and direction are essential. The very successful parents are able to provide continuous, sustained auditory input outside rehabilitative therapy sessions. Ultimately, their children are recipients of intensive, persistent auditory input that enables them to develop residual hearing. The parents are coached and guided by rehabilitation professionals. In my day, less active rehabilitation was performed directly by our parents. The therapy was left to the professionals, who had an opportunity for input only during our therapeutic sessions. Today, children benefit from a more global input throughout the day.

Even though there was less formal instruction by my parents, there was still intensive parental involvement, frequently to my chagrin and resentment. They were overly protective and constantly giving mixed signals: While they told me I was bright enough to achieve, implicit in their obvious concern was their anxiety about whether such achievement was a realistic possibility. The need for more effort from me conflicted with their concern about unduly stressing me in a possibly untenable situation. Their anxiety led me to understand their concerns about my ability to survive and to be self-sufficient as an adult. On one hand, I was told to sit up front in the classroom, which emphasized that I had a hearing loss; but when I didn't hear them at home, I was told, "You're not paying attention," which was essentially a euphemism denying my hearing loss.

Too often the referring physician, whether an otologist or a pediatrician, is unaware of a child's progress with auditory rehabilitation. He or she should be familiar with the milestones the child is attaining under the auspices of a program of a given speech-and-hearing rehabilitation center. There should be a meaningful determination of whether the center has a successful track record in mainstreaming its children. Glossy brochures do not necessarily provide this type of information. Results of auditory rehabilitation vary from center to center or even within a given facility. This may be due to policy, personnel, children, hearing loss, parents, or socioeconomic reasons. Even as a child, I witnessed a tremendous range of professional skill. In retrospect, many aural-rehabilitation professionals were unfocused and were easily manipulated or distracted by me from proceeding with the required therapy.

Some questions the objective referring physician may ask include
- Is the child truly developing language and effective reading to be successfully mainstreamed?
- Are FM units indicated and appropriately used?
- Is there sufficient professional staffing for intensive therapy?
- Are the parents being actively guided to maximize their participation at home for optimal aural rehabilitation?

If effective progress is lacking, then a second or third opinion should be sought to determine why this is occurring and if alternative strategies would be more effective. The pediatrician or primary physician should encourage the parents to probe for a more efficacious rehabilitation if there is insufficient progress. I cannot overemphasize how important it is for the pediatrician to be the child's advocate to ensure that he or she has an optimal chance for aural rehabilitation from a center that has successful experience. If the child's rehabilitation is not progressing, then there has to be an intensive effort with further analysis and/or other opinions to determine why before going on to alternative modalities, eg, total or sign-language communication.

As the child's advocate, the pediatrician should appreciate that language acquisition, along with other developmental milestones, occurs maximally during the critical first few years of childhood. The physician should be aggressive in initiating rehabilitation as early as possible and then closely monitor the child's progress. I have also found that parents are grateful for this purposeful guidance because they finally anticipate a possible solution to their child's hearing loss instead of being frustrated and overwhelmed by their inability to achieve any progress. Empowered with a means to achieve aural and speech rehabilitation for their children, these confident parents also impart a stronger sense of security and a nurturing encouragement to the children.

In my case, high-school education was supplemented with private tutoring in the weaker subjects. Mathematics was difficult because it was awkward to follow this "blackboard" subject with the teacher facing away from me, so that I could not read his or her lips. Even when I was able to see the teacher, following the blackboard activity and "hearing" by reading the teacher's lips at the same time was very difficult. I found prereading mathematics textbooks nonproductive because the subject did not lend itself to prose explanation. My grades were inconsistent and I was characterized as an underachiever.

It is interesting to recall that science was attractive because of its direct potential application to my hearing loss: I used to contemplate how an electromagnetic flux could stimulate the auditory-nerve fibers. In retrospect, this interest in auditory function separated me from my peers: At that time, I was quietly proud of my knowledge, even though it was quite limited. Nevertheless, it was my unique sphere of accomplishment.

Foreign languages were deemed too difficult, and I did find it inordinately frustrating to follow Spanish during a preliminary conversational trial period in the eighth grade. Others were building upon what they heard in the classroom, in contrast to the limited auditory input I was receiving in this listening situation. Thus, it was ultimately deemed that I should learn Latin; in retrospect, this was my good fortune, as it gave me a better understanding of language.

After I graduated from high school at age 18, my parents sent me to Spain for 3 months, where I lived with a Spanish family and attended a Spanish class during the day. There were three students in my class and I was drilled intensively for about 3 hours a day, but no differently from the two normal-hearing students. By the end of this period, I was able to speak Spanish, had become aware of the inchoate aural rhythm and sensation of Spanish words, and also found myself dreaming in Spanish. Although I was aware of dormant auditory activity, I was still a better lip reader than a listener of the language. My minimal listening skills have atrophied, and my current ability to follow Spanish is nil.

Nevertheless, this experience indicated to me that there still was a latent auditory function that could not be activated without a concentrated effort to use my residual hearing. This experience has made me feel that many hearing-impaired children do have a residual auditory substrate that can be used if there is an intensive effort to reach it, especially during the first few years of life.

I believe that the major role for today's pediatrician is to maintain vigilance to see that maximum auditory function is attained, whether it requires resolution of middle ear effusion superimposed on normal or abnormal sensorineural hearing or aural amplification for sensorineural hearing loss (SNHL and/or conductive) appropriately identified in the early months of life, and to see that access to optimal rehabilitation is achieved as early as possible. It is necessary to keep probing and pushing for optimal auditory rehabilitation by encouraging parents to determine if rehabilitation is enabling the child to achieve appropriate milestones.

My challenges in college and in medical school were academically similar. Since I was being "vocationally rehabilitated," a notetaker's services were funded by the state. My classmates certainly found his services helpful. Today, I understand that the New York University medical class collectively funds a notetaker service for everyone in the class. It's nice to know that I was a leader in medical education.

During medical school and my residency, I used assistive listening devices such as amplified stethoscopes and a telephone-activated reading light over the bed so that I could hear the phone ring when I was on call at the hospital. Today, in the operating room, I usually can hear my colleagues, since we are close to each other over the operative site. Because I have stayed in academic medicine, I have residents who are my "ears" to bring me information from beyond the immediate operative field—from the anesthesiologist, the circulating nurse, and the intercom. Teaching conferences are generally no problem if one person is talking and satisfactory illumination is present. Histopathologic presentations, especially those by people with accents, are problematic. The extraneous light from an overhead projector allows me to see the radiologist and follow the presentation. In essence, my hearing loss does not preclude a practice in my specialty, even though I've had to use alternative strategies to help myself and my patients.

While I have touched on some aspects of my "development" and my career, it is obvious that much of my progress was due to the intensive efforts and support of others, including my family, auditory-rehabilitation professionals, teachers, and, more recently, faculty mentors, especially during medical school and residency.

I hope that after this sojourn, the primary-care physician not only will understand the necessity of early diagnosis and therapeutic intervention, but also will appreciate his or her long-term role in providing continued guidance, encouragement, monitoring, and assessment of the patient's progress. The pediatrician should also be convinced that early intervention and later sustained involvement will indeed be fruitful for patients and their families.

Session VIII— Advocacy

Guidelines for Physicians Who Treat Hearing-Impaired Children

Bonnie P. Tucker, JD

Points To Recall:
- *The pediatrician's attitude toward deafness will have significant impact on the parents.*
- *Resources are available (**Appendix B**).*
- *Legislation is coming into effect with which the pediatrician should be familiar.*

A pediatrician, audiologist, or otolaryngologist is usually the person who has the unenviable job of telling parents that their "perfect" baby or child—who in most cases has no visible sign of any impairment—is hearing-impaired. This is a tremendous responsibility, because the manner in which this information is imparted to parents often sets the stage for the child's upbringing. If the physician presents the child's hearing impairment as an insoluble tragedy, the parents will treat it as an insoluble tragedy. We have all heard horror stories of doctors saying bluntly to parents, "Your child is profoundly deaf. He will never learn to speak and will be very limited in his ability to perform in this hearing world. You might as well face that right now." Most parents who hear a statement like that from a trusted physician immediately give up. On the other hand, if the doctor states the case matter of factly, not minimizing the gravity of the situation but explaining that there are solutions to the problems that will undoubtedly arise, the parents may be prepared from the onset to work with their child to overcome those problems. Thus, physicians must take precautions to present the fact of their child's hearing loss to parents in the most positive manner possible.

Having informed parents about the *fact* of their child's deafness, the pediatrician or otolaryngologist must now explain the *meaning* of the deafness. This is an even more difficult task. Parents must, of course, be informed that since their child cannot hear, the child will not obtain information or learn to speak through "normal" channels, but will require comprehensive training to allow him or her to receive and impart information through other means. Parents should be given a brief overview of the two basic philosophies and goals of training deaf children: 1) the oral or auditory-verbal approach, which focuses on the use of residual hearing and/or lip reading and seeks to prepare deaf children to live primarily in the hearing world, and 2) the total-communication approach, which focuses primarily on sign language and preparing deaf children to live in a "deaf society." In addition, parents should immediately be steered to a qualified audiologist to have their child fitted with hearing aids and should be assisted in obtaining audiologic *training* for their child. In this regard, physicians should be aware of the following facts:

1) The hearing of a child or infant of *any* age can be tested.
2) Hearing-impaired infants can (and should, if possible) wear hearing aids.
3) Initial testing often does not reflect the thresholds of hearing (test may show the hearing loss to be greater than it actually is).
4) Today, hearing aids are more powerful and have greater capabilities than ever before. Cochlear implants are available for children 2 years of age and older.
5) Even severely and profoundly deaf children can learn to use hearing aids (and their remaining hearing) to acquire language and speech. There are few totally deaf children. Even very limited hearing can become functional with proper habilitation.
6) Hearing tests and hearing-aid evaluations do not infallibly indicate or predict the degree to which a child will learn to use hearing aids.
7) If remaining hearing and hearing aids are to be used, the child should be in a program that strengthens the weakest sense (hearing) rather than the strongest sense (eg, vision, via sign language).
8) Hearing aids alone, without concurrent training, are of no practical assistance.
9) The choice of whether to a) teach a child to speak, use his or her residual hearing, and lip read, or b) teach a child to sign, will determine whether the child becomes part of a culturally distinct deaf subculture or part of mainstream society.

The physician should provide the parents with a list of agencies and organizations in their state or city that will assist them in obtaining necessary services and information. At a minimum, parents should be given the phone numbers of the national offices of the Alexander Graham Bell Association for the Deaf in Washington, DC (202/337-5220), and the National Association of the Deaf in Maryland (301/587-6282). These two organizations can refer parents to local agencies that espouse their respective philosophies (oralism and total communication), and should be able to provide parents with informative books, pamphlets, and/or videos. In addition, **Appendix B** lists agencies in the various states and Canada that parents may contact for assistance and information.

Physicians should encourage parents to ask applicable agencies and organizations for the names of parents of other deaf children—who can usually serve as invaluable resources in addition to providing empathetic ears—and of deaf people in the community—who may be the best source of real-life information about what deafness means (and who may well be the first deaf people the parents meet).

In addition to providing parents with basic information about deafness and sources of assistance, it would be helpful if pediatricians and otolaryngologists had some general knowledge of the federal laws that require states receiving federal funds for educational programs to provide educational assistance to all children with disabilities from birth through the age of 21 years. Parents need to know that there are laws to assist them in obtaining necessary services for their deaf children, so they may take advantage of the services available. Following is a very brief overview of the significant law in this area:

Federal Legislation for Educational Assistance
For Children 0 to 3 Years of Age

The Education for All Handicapped Children Act (EAHCA) (now called the Individuals With Disabilities Education Act—IDEA) was enacted in the late 1970s to ensure that children with disabilities were provided with appropriate educational services at state expense. In 1986, Part H of the EAHCA [20 U.S.C.A. §§ 1471-1485 (1990)] was enacted to protect the interests of disabled infants and toddlers.

Part H of the EAHCA creates a discretionary program to assist states in planning coordinated, comprehensive, multidisciplinary, interagency programs that provide early-intervention services for disabled infants from birth to 3 years of age. States may opt into this program, and thereby receive federal funds for providing early-intervention services to handicapped infants and toddlers, by complying with a 5-year program for the development of services for such children. Basically, a state has 5 years to develop a program for early-intervention services for disabled infants and toddlers. By the beginning of the 4th year, the state must have in place a system for providing services; by the beginning of the 5th year, the state must make the services available to all eligible infants and toddlers. States must designate a lead agency that is responsible for planning and operating this comprehensive system, and each governor must appoint an Interagency Coordinating Council (ICC) to advise and assist the state's lead agency. All 50 states have opted into this program. Although most states have assigned as the lead agency their department of education or health, a few states have designated other agencies (Arizona, for example, has designated the Department of Economic Security). But a parent who wants to contact the applicable agency can always call the governor's office and ask for the number of the state's ICC.

The 1st "year" of the 5-year planning period was July 1, 1987 through September 30, 1988. Thus, the 5th year—when early-intervention services must be provided to disabled infants and toddlers—is the beginning of the 1992-1993 fiscal year (in some cases, the beginning of the 1991-1992 fiscal year). By that time, disabled infants and toddlers who are experiencing developmental delays or have a diagnosed physical or mental condition that has a high probability of resulting in developmental delay—which includes hearing-impaired children—must be provided with early-intervention services. "Early-intervention services" under Part H are defined as developmental services provided under public supervision that are designed to meet the child's needs in physical development, cognitive development, language and speech development, psychosocial development, and/or the development of self-help skills. These services may include

> (i) family training, counseling and home visits; (ii) special instruction; (iii) speech pathology and audiology; (iv) occupational therapy; (v) physical therapy; (vi) psychological services; (vii) case management services; (viii) medical services only for diagnostic or evaluation purposes; (ix) early identification, screening, and assessment services; (x) health services necessary to enable the infant or toddler to benefit from the other early intervention services.... [20 U.S.C.A. § 1472(E) (1990)].

While the states have the option of charging parents for some of these services, such as speech and language services, the charges must be based on a schedule of sliding fees, and no child may be denied services due to the family's inability to pay.

Under Part H, the family of each eligible infant or toddler must be provided with a case manager, who is responsible for helping the parents obtain the services and assistance they require and are entitled to under the act. The parents may not be charged for these case-management services. Case managers are required to coordinate evaluations and assessments for the child, assist families in identifying available service providers, coordinate and monitor the delivery of services, inform families of the availability of advocacy services, and facilitate the development of a transition plan to preschool services when the child reaches the age of 3 years. Case managers are required to work with the family to develop an "individualized family service plan" (IFSP) each year that identifies short- and long-term goals for the child and the family.

The focus of Part H is early intervention. Congress recognized that early intervention enhances the development of disabled infants, minimizes their potential for developmental delay, reduces overall educational costs, enhances the capacity of families to meet the special needs of their disabled infants and toddlers, minimizes the likelihood of the institutionalization of such children, and maximizes the potential for disabled people to live independently in society. Early-intervention services will be especially important to families of hearing-impaired children, since the early provision of auditory, speech, and language training is crucial to prevent irremediable loss of significant language development. Moreover, Part H also requires each state to establish and maintain a central directory containing information about public and private early-intervention services, resources, and experts available in the state and professional and other groups (including parent-support groups and advocacy associations) that provide assistance to eligible children and their families. This central directory, if properly developed, should be of enormous value to both physicians and parents.

Because most parents today discover the fact of their child's hearing impairment while the child is still an infant, it is important that parents be informed about Part H so they may seek appropriate state assistance. The National Information Center for Children and Youth With Handicaps (PO Box 1492, Washington, DC 20013) publishes a free pamphlet—available on request—that provides an overview of Part H.

For Children, Youth, and Young Adults 3 to 21 Years of Age

Part B of the IDEA [20 U.S.C.A. §§ 1400-1471 (1990)] requires each state that receives federal assistance for educational programs to provide each disabled resident from the ages of 3 to 21 years a free, appropriate, public education (FAPE). The focus of Part B is on providing an educational program that meets the individual needs of each disabled child. Thus, each year educators must meet with the parents of every hearing-impaired child in their district to plan an individualized education program (IEP) that meets the unique needs of that child. In addition, Part B requires that every disabled child be educated in the least restrictive environment possible for that child. For some hearing-impaired children, that will be a mainstream program; for others, it will be a special oral program; for still others, it will be a special total-communication program.

Part B of the IDEA is enormously complex. Much litigation has arisen over its various provisions since the law was implemented. For the purposes of the physician, however, it is only important to have a general awareness of Part B, so that parents can be informed that the law exists.

Part B was amended to create enhanced incentives for states to provide an FAPE to all disabled children between 3 and 6 years of age. States that do not do so will lose enormous sums of money (including preschool grant money, funds generated under Part B of the state-plan formula for 3- to 5-year-olds, and designated discretionary grants). Because services such as speech and language training are so important to preschool hearing-impaired children, parents should be informed about this law and told to contact the state's department of education to determine what services are available for their preschool children. Parents who are dissatisfied with the services provided should request that their school district provide them with a due process hearing. The parents may wish to contact the Center for Law in the Public Interest or a similar state agency and request assistance. As a last resort, the parents may want to hire an attorney and file suit in federal court.

Significant Legislation

Two other subjects that should be addressed are early identification of hearing loss and the Americans With Disabilities Act (ADA) of 1990.

Early Identification of Hearing Loss

It is crucial that children with prelingual hearing losses be identified as early as possible so that the accompanying speech, language, and educational difficulties may be dealt with immediately. The American Academy of Otolaryngology—Head and Neck Surgery has stated that "[b]y using a concept of high-risk factors to identify children likely to be hearing-impaired, and following up with state-of-the-art computerized hearing testing, around 75% of all hearing losses should be detected."[*] To that end, at least 17 states[**] have implemented legislation providing for some form of mandatory neonatal hearing screening—to determine which infants are at high risk of being born with hearing losses. At least an additional 12 states[†] that do not have legislative mandates have addressed the issue at the state level. The types of screening either mandated or recommended vary widely. Basically, however, they follow two approaches.

The first approach involves compilation of a high-risk registry. High-risk infants are identified and placed on the registry through either information provided when their birth certificate forms are completed or information obtained during in-hospital chart reviews completed by hospital personnel. Subsequently, parents of infants at risk for hearing loss are notified of that fact and given information about where to go for testing. Some follow-up is conducted to determine whether the infants were, in fact, tested.

The second approach is an in-hospital approach, in which high-risk infants are identified and provided with audiologic screening before discharge. Infants who do not pass the screening or who are found to be at risk for progressive hearing loss are retested 3 to 6 months after being discharged.

Infant-hearing screening programs vary widely in form and substance between states. Some obviously are more effective than others. In addition, other states are currently in the discussion or planning stages with respect to developing such programs. Physicians who often treat children with hearing losses may want to become involved in the planning or implementation of an infant-screening program in their state. Those who do should contact Susan Coffman at the Alexander Graham Bell Association for the Deaf in Washington, DC, or Moira De Wilde at the American Academy of Otolaryngology—Head and Neck Surgery in Alexandria, Virginia (703/836-4444), and ask for a copy of the materials prepared by the Joint Committee on Early Identification of Hearing Loss.

Americans With Disabilities Act of 1990

Under the recently enacted ADA, by January 26, 1992, physicians must make accommodations for disabled people, to allow disabled people to benefit to the same extent as nondisabled patients from their services. For example, a physician might be required to provide an

---

[*]Joint Committee on Infant Hearing Screening, Statement of Need (Sept 26, 1990) (on file with author)
[**]Arizona, California, Connecticut, Florida, Georgia, Hawaii, Kansas, Kentucky, Maryland, Massachusetts, Mississippi, New Jersey, Ohio, Oklahoma, Rhode Island, Virginia, West Virginia
[†]Alaska, Arkansas, Colorado, Delaware, Michigan, Montana, New Mexico, North Dakota, Pennsylvania, Utah, Wisconsin, Wyoming

interpreter so that a deaf patient whose primary language is American Sign Language can converse with the doctor and staff. Moreover, physicians must remove structural, architectural, and communication barriers in their offices to the extent that such removal is "easily accomplishable and able to be carried out without much difficulty or expense." In a large office facility, for example, one or more doorways might have to be widened so that the waiting room and some patient rooms are accessible to people in wheelchairs. A physician may not refuse to treat a patient whom he or she would otherwise treat because the patient requires an accommodation. The Department of Justice promulgated regulations dealing with this section of the ADA in July 1991. The regulations will provide some specificity with respect to the obligation of physicians and other owners and operators of places of public accommodation under the ADA.

Discussion

Dr Hart: A neonatal screening program was initiated in Arizona that did not emanate from a university, department of health, department of education, or the Department of Economic Security. It started from grass roots and included physicians from many different disciplines, audiologists, hearing-aid dispensers, the Arizona School for the Deaf and Blind, and university personnel. The program was officially enabled by the Arizona legislature, which has seen that if money is wisely spent initially, much more money can be saved at the back end.

We continue to have problems, however, partly because—I think—pediatricians don't have adequate experience, individually, with hearing loss or with deaf children, and partly because we pediatricians are all trained to assume that things will get better, that children will "grow out of it," or that problems will go away.

Appendix A:
Joint Committee on Infant Hearing 1990 Position Statement*

Approved by the American Speech-Language-Hearing Association (ASHA) Legislative Council in November 1990, this position statement was prepared by representatives from ASHA, the American Academy of Otolaryngology—Head and Neck Surgery, American Academy of Pediatrics, Council on Education of the Deaf, and directors of speech and hearing programs in state health and welfare agencies.

I. Background

The early detection of hearing impairment in children is essential in order to initiate the medical and educational intervention critical for developing optimal communication and social skills. In 1982, the Joint Committee on Infant Hearing recommended identifying infants at risk for hearing impairment by means of seven criteria and suggested follow-up audiologic evaluation of these infants until accurate assessments of hearing could be made.[1] In recent years, advances in science and technology have increased the chances for survival of markedly premature and low-birth-weight neonates and other severely compromised newborns. Because moderate to severe sensorineural hearing loss can be confirmed in 2.5% to 5.0% of neonates manifesting any of the previously published risk criteria, auditory screening of at-risk newborns is warranted.[2-5] Those infants who have one or more of the risk factors are considered to be at increased risk for sensorineural hearing loss.

Recent research and new legislation (Public Law 99-457) suggest the need for expansion and clarification of the 1982 criteria. This 1991 statement expands the risk criteria and makes recommendations for the identification and management of hearing-impaired neonates and infants. The Joint Committee recognizes that the performance characteristics of these new risk factors are not presently known; further study and critical evaluation of the risk criteria are therefore encouraged. The protocols recommended by the Committee are considered optimal and are based on both clinical experience and current research findings. The Committee recognizes, however, that the recommended protocols may not be appropriate for all institutions and that modifications in screening approaches will be necessary to accommodate the specific needs of a given facility. Such factors as cost and availability of equipment, personnel, and follow-up services are important considerations in the development of a screening program.[6]

II. Identification

A. Risk Criteria: Neonates (birth to 28 days)
The risk factors that identify those neonates who are at risk for sensorineural hearing impairment include the following:
   1. Family history of congenital or delayed-onset childhood sensorineural impairment.

*Reprinted from *AAO-HNS Bulletin*, March 1991, with permission

2. Congenital infection known or suspected to be associated with sensorineural hearing impairment such as toxoplasmosis, syphilis, rubella, cytomegalovirus, and herpes.
3. Craniofacial anomalies including morphologic abnormalities of the pinna and ear canal, absent philtrum, low hairline, etc.
4. Birth weight less than 1500 g (< 3.3 lb).
5. Hyperbilirubinemia at a level exceeding indication for exchange transfusion.
6. Ototoxic medications including but not limited to the aminoglycosides used for more than 5 days (eg, gentamicin, tobramycin, kanamycin, streptomycin) and loop diuretics used in combination with aminoglycosides.
7. Bacterial meningitis.
8. Severe depression at birth, which may include infants with Apgar scores of 0 to 3 at 5 minutes or those who fail to initiate spontaneous respiration by 10 minutes or those with hypotonia persisting to 2 hours of age.
9. Prolonged mechanical ventilation for a duration equal to or greater than 10 days (eg, persistent pulmonary hypertension).
10. Stigmata or other findings associated with a syndrome known to include sensorineural hearing loss (eg, Waardenburg or Usher syndrome).

B. Risk Criteria: Infants (29 days to 2 years)
The factors that identify those infants who are at risk for sensorineural hearing impairment include the following:
1. Parent/caregiver concern regarding hearing, speech, language, and/or developmental delay.
2. Bacterial meningitis.
3. Neonatal risk factors that may be associated with progressive sensorineural hearing loss (eg, cytomegalovirus, prolonged mechanical ventilation, and inherited disorders).
4. Head trauma, especially with either longitudinal or transverse fracture of the temporal bone.
5. Stigmata or other findings associated with syndromes known to include sensorineural hearing loss (eg, Waardenburg or Usher syndrome).
6. Ototoxic medications including but not limited to the aminoglycosides used for more than 5 days (eg, gentamicin, tobramycin, kanamycin, streptomycin) and loop diuretics used in combination with aminoglycosides.
7. Children with neurodegenerative disorders such as neurofibromatosis, myoclonic epilepsy, Werdnig-Hoffmann disease, Tay-Sachs disease, infantile Gaucher disease, Niemann-Pick disease, any metachromatic leukodystrophy, or any infantile demyelinating neuropathy.
8. Childhood infectious diseases known to be associated with sensorineural hearing loss (eg, mumps, measles).

III. Audiologic Screening Recommendations for Neonates and Infants

A. Neonates
Neonates who manifest one or more items on the risk criteria should be screened, preferably under the supervision of an audiologist. Optimally, screening should be completed prior to discharge from the newborn nursery but no later than 3 months of age. The initial screening should include measurement of the auditory brain-stem response (ABR).[7] Behavioral testing of newborn infants' hearing has high false-positive and false-negative rates and is not universally recommended. Because some false-positive results can occur with ABR screening, ongoing assessment and observation of the infant's auditory behavior is

recommended during the early stages of intervention. If the infant is discharged prior to screening, or if ABR screening under audiologic supervision is not available, the child ideally should be referred for ABR testing by 3 months of age but never later than 6 months of age.

The acoustic stimulus for ABR screening should contain energy in the frequency region important for speech recognition. Clicks are the most commonly used signal for eliciting the ABR and contain energy in the speech frequency region.[7] Pass criterion for ABR screening is a response from each ear at intensity levels 40 dB nHL or less. Transducers designed to reduce the probability of ear canal collapse are recommended.

If consistent electrophysiologic responses are detected at appropriate sound levels, then the screening process will be considered complete except in those cases where there is a probability of progressive hearing loss (eg, family history of delayed onset, degenerative disease, meningitis, intrauterine infections, or infants who had chronic lung disease, pulmonary hypertension, or who received medications in doses likely to be ototoxic). If the results of an initial screening of an infant manifesting any risk criteria are equivocal, then the infant should be referred for general medical, otologic, and audiologic follow-up.

B. Infants

Infants who exhibit one or more items on the risk criteria should be screened as soon as possible but no later than 3 months after the child has been identified as at risk. For infants less than 6 months of age, ABR screening (see II A.) is recommended. For infants older than 6 months, behavioral testing using a conditioned response or ABR testing is an appropriate approach. Infants who fail the screen should be referred for a comprehensive audiologic evaluation. This evaluation may include ABR, behavioral testing (6 months), and acoustic immittance measures.[7]

IV. Early Intervention for Hearing-Impaired Infants and Their Families

When hearing loss is identified, early intervention services should be provided, in accordance with Public Law 99-457. Early intervention services under PL 99-457 may commence before the completion of the evaluation and assessment if the following conditions are met: a) parental consent is obtained, b) an interim individualized family service plan (IFSP) is developed, and c) the full initial evaluation process is completed within 45 days of referral.

The interim IFSP should include the following:

A. The name of the case manager who will be responsible for both implementation of the interim IFSP and coordination with other agencies and persons;

B. The early intervention services that have been determined to be needed immediately by the child and the child's family.

These immediate early intervention services should include the following:

1. Evaluation by a physician with expertise in the management of early-childhood otologic disorders.

2. Evaluation by an audiologist with expertise in the assessment of young children, to determine the type, degree, and configuration of the hearing loss, and to recommend assistive communication devices appropriate to the child's needs (eg, hearing aids, personal FM systems, vibrotactile aids).

3. Evaluation by a speech-language pathologist, teacher of the hearing-impaired, audiologist, or other professional with expertise in the assessment of communication skills in hearing-impaired children, to develop a program of early intervention consistent with the needs of the child and preferences of the

family. Such intervention would be cognizant of and sensitive to cultural values inherent in familial deafness.

4. Family education, counseling, and guidance, including home visits and parent support groups to provide families with information, child-management skills, and emotional support consistent with the needs of the child and family and their culture.

5. Special instruction that includes:

   a. the design and implementation of learning environments and activities that promote the child's development and communication skills;

   b. curriculum planning that integrates and coordinates multidisciplinary personnel and resources so that intended outcomes of the IFSP are achieved; and

   c. ongoing monitoring of the child's hearing status and amplification needs and development of auditory skills.

V. Future Considerations for Risk Criteria

Because of the dynamic changes occurring in neonatal-prenatal medicine, the committee recognizes that forthcoming research may result in the need for revision of the 1991 risk register. For example, the committee has concerns about the possible ototoxic effects on the fetus from maternal drug abuse; however, present data are insufficient to determine whether the fetus or neonate is at risk for hearing loss. In addition, yet-to-be-developed medications may have ototoxic effects on neonates and infants. Therefore, the committee advises clinicians to keep apprised of published reports demonstrating correlations between maternal drug abuse and ototoxicity and between future antimicrobial agents and ototoxicity. Clinicians should also take into account the possible interactive effects of multiple medications administered simultaneously. Finally, the committee recommends that the position statement be examined every 3 years for possible revision.

References

1. Joint Committee on Infant Hearing: Position statement. *ASHA* 1982;24:1017.
2. Hosford-Dunn H, Johnson S, Simmons B, et al: Infant hearing screening: Program implementation and validation. *Ear Hear* 1987;8:12.
3. Jacobson J, Morehouse R: A comparison of auditory brainstem response and behavioral screening in high risk and normal newborn infants. *Ear Hear* 1984;5:245.
4. Mahoney TM, Eichwald JG: The ups and "downs" of high risk hearing screening: The Utah statewide program, in Gerkin KP, Amochaev A (eds): *Semin Hear* 1987;8:155.
5. Stein L, Ozdamar O, Kraus N, Paton J: Follow-up of infants screened by auditory brainstem response in the neonatal intensive care unit. *J Pediatr* 1983;63:447.
6. Turner RG: Analysis of recommended guidelines for infant hearing screening. *ASHA* 1990;32:57.
7. American Speech-Language-Hearing Association: Guidelines for audiologic screening of newborn infants who are at-risk for hearing impairment. *ASHA* 1989;31(3):89.

Appendix B: Information Services February 1991

Compiled by Bonnie P. Tucker, JD

Alabama

Alexander Graham Bell Association for the Deaf
Betty Faircloth, Chapter President
315 Clanton Ave
Montgomery, AL 36104

Alexander Graham Bell Association for the Deaf
Children's Rights Coordinators
Ronald Evelsizer, EdD
Speech and Hearing Center
University of Alabama
PO Box 1903
Tuscaloosa, AL 35487-1903
Tel: 205-339-2633 (home)
   205-348-7131 (work)

Sarah Spurlock McLain
716 Sanders Rd
Birmingham, AL 35226
Tel: 205-823-4256 (home)
   205-252-1766 (work)

Deaf CONTACT
3224 Executive Park Circle
Mobile, AL 36606
Tel: 205-342-3333 (voice)
   205-343-4555 (TDD*)

Janice Capilouto Center for the Deaf
1521 Mulberry St
Montgomery, AL 36106
Tel: 205-264-4533 (voice/TDD)

Arizona

Alexander Graham Bell Association for the Deaf
Peggy Shapiro, Chapter President
PO Box 922
Mesa, AZ 85201
Tel: 602-491-2082 (home)

Alexander Graham Bell Association for the Deaf
Children's Rights Coordinator
Maxine Turnbull
2453 E LaJolla Dr
Tempe, AZ 85282
Tel: 602-820-6657 (home)
   602-820-8817 (work)

Council for the Hearing Impaired
Director: Stuart R. Brackney, MA
1300 W Washington
Phoenix, AZ 85007
Tel: 602-255-3323 (voice/TDD)

Listen, Inc
Maxine Turnbull, Director
2453 E LaJolla Dr
Tempe, AZ 85282
Tel: 602-820-8817

Arkansas

Alexander Graham Bell Association for the Deaf
Children's Rights Coordinators
Nan Ellen East
11 Tanglewood Lane
Little Rock, AR 72202
Tel: 501-664-2379 (home)
   501-371-2171 (work)

Sally Neuner
#40 9th Fairway Loop
Maumelle, AR 72118
Tel: 501-851-1150

Arkansas Association for Hearing-Impaired Children
Lynn Coates
2214 N Palm
Little Rock, AR 72207

Office for the Deaf & Hearing Impaired
4324 W Markham
Little Rock, AR 72205
Tel: 501-371-1922 (voice)
   501-371-1924 (TDD)

---
*Telecommunications Device for the Deaf

Deaf Outreach Center
4601 W Markham
Little Rock, AR 72205
Tel: 501-371-7647 (voice)
 501-371-7667 (TDD)

California

Alexander Graham Bell Association for the Deaf
Charlie Lane, Chapter President
Apt 4
6081 Claremont Ave
Oakland, CA 94618
Tel: 217-359-7887

Alexander Graham Bell Association for the Deaf
Children's Rights Coordinators
Jean Ching
1068 Sladky Ave
Mountain View, CA 94040
Tel: 415-967-4579 (home)
 415-856-0855 (work)

Dr Jeri Traub
Division of Special Education and Rehabilitative Services
Sweeney Hall 204
San Jose State University
San Jose, CA 95192-0078
Tel: 408-920-2201 (home)
 408-924-3678 (work)

Sally Wood
433 E Meadow Dr
Palo Alto, CA 94306
Tel: 415-493-0609 (home)
 415-856-0855 (work)

Cynthia Runstrom
6311 Sierra Elena
Irvine, CA 92715
Tel: 714-854-7582

Cathy Walsh
11089 Viacha Dr
San Diego, CA 92124
Tel: 619-560-4604 (home)
 619-694-2001 (work)

ECHO Center
Fay Shutsky
3430 McManus Ave
Culver City, CA 90232
Tel: 213-838-2442

Jean Weigarten Peninsula Oral School for the Deaf
Leahea Grammatico
2525 Buena Vista Ave
Belmont, CA 94002
Tel: 415-593-1848

John Tracy Clinic
Dr James Garrity
806 West Adams Blvd
Los Angeles, CA 90007
Tel: 213-748-5481

Oralingua School
Etta L. Fisher
7056 S Washington Ave
Whittier, CA 90602
Tel: 213-945-8391
 714-523-4570

Valley Advocacy & Communication Center for the Deaf and Hearing Impaired (VACC)
441 W Olive St, Suite 3
Fresno, CA 93728
Tel: 209-486-8222

Greater Los Angeles Council on Deafness, Inc (GLAD)
616 S Westmoreland Ave
2nd Floor
Los Angeles, CA 90005
Tel: 213-383-2220 (voice/TDD)

University of California-Irvine, Deafness Center
101 City Dr S, Building 53
Orange, CA 92668
Tel: 714-634-6021

NorCal Center on Deafness
2400 Glendale Lane, Suite F
Sacramento, CA 95825
Tel: 916-486-8570 (voice/TDD)

Deaf Community Services of San Diego, Inc
3788 Park Blvd
San Diego, CA 92103
Tel: 619-692-0932 (voice/TDD)

Hearing Society for the Bay Area, Inc
1428 Bush St
San Francisco, CA 94109
Tel: 415-775-5700 (voice)
 415-776-3323 (TDD)

Colorado

Alexander Graham Bell Association for the Deaf
Children's Rights Coordinator
Meredith Schmidt
1196 E Bates Parkway
Englewood, CO 80110
Tel: 303-789-5482

Pikes Peak Center on Deafness
1322 N Academy, Suite 104
Colorado Springs, CO 80909
Tel: 303-591-2777 (voice)
 303-591-2333 (TDD)

Center on Deafness
2250 Eaton St
Edgewater, CO 80214
Tel: 303-235-0015 (voice/TDD)

Connecticut

Alexander Graham Bell Association for the Deaf
John Garvin, Chapter President
54 Stratton Dr
Chesho, CT 06410
Tel: 203-271-1218 (home-voice/TDD)
    203-378-8281 (work)
    203-381-0543 (work-FAX)

Alexander Graham Bell Association for the Deaf
Children's Rights Coordinator
Maurine Kessler
22 Hamlin Dr
West Hartford, CT 06117
Tel: 203-523-7745 (home)
    203-397-4573 (work)

Connecticut Commission on the Deaf & Hearing Impaired
40 Woodland St
Hartford, CT 06105
Tel: 203-566-7414 (voice/TDD)

Newington Children's Hospital Speech Pathology & Audiology
181 E Cedar St
Newington, CT 06111
Tel: 203-667-5320

Hearing Improvement Center
10 N Main St
West Hartford, CT 06107
Tel: 203-232-5947 (voice)
    203-236-5948 (TDD)

Florida

Alexander Graham Bell Association for the Deaf
Irene Nardandrea, Chapter President
733 NW 41 Terrace
Deerfield Beach, FL 33442
Tel: 904-738-3236

Alexander Graham Bell Association for the Deaf
Children's Rights Coordinators
Kyle Aguero
6532 SW 106th Ave
Miami, FL 33173
Tel: 305-279-5951 (home)
    305-666-3446 (work)

Joan C. Rollins Bellows
Ralph J. Baudhuin Oral School of Nova University
3375 SW 75th Ave
Fort Lauderdale, FL 33314
Tel: 305-475-7324

Judy Heavner, PhD
Program Specialist, Hearing Impaired
Florida Dept of Education
Division of Public Schools
W.V. Knott Building
Tallahassee, FL 32399-0400
Tel: 904-488-3103

Joe Kulakowski
1709 Montgomery St
Holly Hill, FL 32017
Tel: 904-673-9167 (home)
    904-254-3844 ext 183 (work)

Dr Marya Mavilya
416 Surfside Blvd
Surfside, FL 33154
Tel: 305-865-2995

Linda C. Strauss, EdD
8631 NW 82nd St
Tamorac, FL 33321
Tel: 305-720-1740 (home)
    305-445-5188 (work)

McCord-Bolesta Speech and Hearing Center
Ethel Denney Bolesta
4016 Estrelle, PO Box 10934
Tampa, FL 33679
Tel: 813-251-6445

Ralph J. Baudhuin Oral School of Nova University
Dr Susan E. Talpins
3375 SW 75th Ave
Fort Lauderdale, FL 33314
Tel: 305-475-7324

Deaf Services Bureau, Inc
4800 W Flagler St, Suite 213
Miami, FL 33134
Tel: 305-444-2266 (voice)
    305-444-2211 (TDD)

Deaf Service Center
4000 W Buffalo Ave, Suite 186
Tampa, FL 33614
Tel: 813-272-3370 (voice)
    813-876-3215 (TDD)

Georgia

The Atlanta Speech School
Dot Grigonis
3160 Northside Parkway, NW
Atlanta, GA 30327
Tel: 404-233-5332

Illinois

Alexander Graham Bell Association for the Deaf
Susan Berlow, Chapter President
150 E Huron, Suite 906
Chicago, IL 60611
Tel: 312-337-8060

Alexander Graham Bell Association for the Deaf
Children's Rights Coordinators
Ann Wilcox Bleuer
PO Box 1099
Park Ridge, IL 60068

Mary Ann Lachman
7702 Davis
Morton Grove, IL 60053
Tel: 312-965-7735

Lutheran Child & Family Services, Hearing-Impaired Program
333 W Lake St
Addison, IL 60101
Tel: 312-628-6448 (voice)
 312-782-6555 (TDD)

Chicago Hearing Society
10 W Jackson St, 4th Floor
Chicago, IL 60604
Tel: 312-939-6888 (voice)
 312-427-2166 (TDD)

Northwestern University Hearing Clinics
303 E Chicago Ave
Chicago, IL 60611
Tel: 312-908-8107

Indiana

Alexander Graham Bell Association for the Deaf
Lorraine Kisselburgh, Chapter President
612 N Salisbury
West Lafayette, IN 47906
Tel: 317-743-6106

June Knight Shassere
4491 Washington Blvd
Indianapolis, IN 46205
Tel: 317-926-3015

Alexander Graham Bell Association for the Deaf
Children's Rights Coordinator
Mary Boucher
6240 Newberry Rd, Apt 805
Indianapolis, IN 46256
Tel: 317-841-9853

Deaf Social Service Agency for the Tri-State, Inc
901 W Virginia St
Evansville, IN 47710
Tel: 812-425-2726 (voice)
 812-425-2841 (TDD)

Community Services for the Deaf
445 N Pennsylvania St, Suite 811
Indianapolis, IN 46204
Tel: 317-637-3947 (voice/TDD)

HEAR Indiana
June Knight Shassere
4491 Washington Blvd
Indianapolis, IN 46205
Tel: 317-926-3015

Iowa

Deaf Services of Iowa
Iowa State Department of Health
Lucas State Office Building
Des Moines, IA 50319
Tel: 515-281-3164 (voice/TDD)

Kansas

Alexander Graham Bell Association for the Deaf
Children's Rights Coordinator
Deborah Hammond
Rt 1, Box 142
Manchester, KS 67463

Kansas Commission for the Deaf and Hearing Impaired
2700 W 6th St
Biddle Building, 1st Floor
Topeka, KS 66606
Tel: 913-296-2874
(1-800-432-0698 in KS only)
 (voice/TDD)

Kentucky

Alexander Graham Bell Association for the Deaf
Rhonda Dean, Chapter President
4403 Windy Oaks Rd
Louisville, KY 40241
Tel: 502-636-2084

Alexander Graham Bell Association
for the Deaf
Children's Rights Coordinator
Kathy Daniel
Louisville Deaf Oral School
414 W Ormsby Ave
Louisville, KY 40203
Tel: 502-636-2084

Lexington Hearing and Speech Center
Carol Jackson
162 N Ashland Ave
Lexington, KY 40502
Tel: 606-268-4545

**Caprice Industries of
Christian Appalachian Project**
412 Anderson Heights
Stanford, KY 40484
Tel: 606-365-9196

**Caprice Industries of
Christian Appalachian Project**
943 Monticello Rd
Somerset, KY 42501
Tel: 606-679-8438

Louisiana

Alexander Graham Bell Association
for the Deaf
Children's Rights Coordinator
Dr Elizabeth Wilkes
Chinchuba Institute
1131 Barataria Blvd
Marrero, LA 70072
Tel: 504-340-9261

**Deaf Resource and
Communication Center**
721 St Ferdinand St
New Orleans, LA 70117-7395
Tel: 504-949-4413 (voice/TDD)

Maine

Alexander Graham Bell Association
for the Deaf
Children's Rights Coordinator
Karen McCall
Downeast School
100 Moosehead Blvd
Bangor, ME 04401
Tel: 207-945-9366 (home)
   207-947-2925 (work)

Maine Association of the Deaf, Inc
PO Box 1014
Portland, ME 04104
Tel: 207-787-2602 (voice/TDD)

Maryland

Alexander Graham Bell Association
for the Deaf
Children's Rights Coordinators
Sue Griebler
8123 Scott's Level Rd
Baltimore, MD 21208
Tel: 301-655-4750
   301-396-4965

Janie Jackson
Terrace 11
9900 Georgia Ave
Silver Spring, MD 20902
Tel: 301-589-5348

Deaf Referral Services, Inc
3700 Greenspring Ave
Baltimore, MD 21211
Tel: 301-225-3323 (voice/TDD)

**Family Service Foundation
Institute on Deafness**
7580 Annapolis Rd
Lanham, MD 20706
Tel: 301-459-2121 (voice)
   301-731-6141 (TDD)

Massachusetts

Alexander Graham Bell Association
for the Deaf
Stephanie Joyce, Chapter President
19 Alyssum Dr
Amherst, MA 01002
Tel: 413-253-9805 (home)
   413-584-3450 (work)

Alexander Graham Bell Association
for the Deaf
Children's Rights Coordinators
Karen Gjerdingen
Coordinator, Admissions Office
Clarke School
Round Hill Rd
Northampton, MA 01060-2499
Tel: 413-584-3450

Judy Kates
158 Bianca Rd
Duxbury, MA 02332

Clarke School for the Deaf
Dennis Gjerdingen, President
Round Hill Rd
Northampton, MA 01060-2499
Tel: 413-584-3450 (voice/TDD)
   413-586-2879 (TDD)

Montgomery County Association for Hearing Impaired Children
Susan Russell
PO Box 303
Boston, MA 02101

Massachusetts Office of Deafness
Richard E. Thompson, PhD, Director
20 Park Plaza, Suite 328
Boston, MA 02116
Tel: 617-727-5236 (TDD)

Massachusetts Commission for the Deaf and Hard of Hearing
600 Washington St
Boston, MA 02111
Tel: 617-727-5106 (TDD)
800-882-1155

Michigan

Alexander Graham Bell Association for the Deaf
Kathleen S. Quinn
1710 Gregory
Ypsilanti, MI 48197
Tel: 313-487-2259 (work)
313-483-4825 (home)

Alexander Graham Bell Association for the Deaf
Children's Rights Coordinator
Beth Young
2100 Pontiac Lake Rd
Pontiac, MI 48054
Tel: 313-349-0584 (home)
313-858-2143 (work)

Social Services for the Hearing Impaired
302 E Court St
Flint, MI 48502
Tel: 313-239-3112 (voice/TDD)

Minnesota

Alexander Graham Bell Association for the Deaf
Children's Rights Coordinators
Deirdre Clements
961 Paxton Rd, SW
Rochester, MN 55902
Tel: 507-289-5795

Winifred Northcott, PhD
4510 Cedarwood Rd
Minneapolis, MN 55416
Tel: 612-922-5889

Minnesota Foundation for Better Hearing and Speech
508 Bremer Building
7th and Robert Sts
St Paul, MN 55101
Tel: 612-223-5310 (voice/TDD)

Minnesota Regional Offices of State Services for the Deaf
Northeast Area Regional Services Center
Government Services Building, Suite 710
320 W 2nd St
Duluth, MN 55802
Tel: 218-723-4962 (voice)
218-723-4961 (TDD)

Minnesota Regional Offices of State Services for the Deaf
Northwest Area Regional Services Center
125 W Lincoln Ave, Suite 7
Fergus Falls, MN 56537
Tel: 218-739-7589 (voice/TDD)

Mississippi

Alexander Graham Bell Association for the Deaf
Children's Rights Coordinator
Barbara Hanners, PhD
Speech/Hearing Center
PO Box W-1340
Columbus, MS 39701
Tel: 601-329-7270

Magnolia Speech School, Inc
Charles Gammel, PhD
733 Flag Chapel Rd
Jackson, MS 39209
Tel: 601-922-5530

Golden Triangle CONTACT
PO Box 1304
Columbus, MS 39703-1304
Tel: 601-328-0200

Missouri

Central Institute for the Deaf
Dr Richard G. Stoker, Superintendent
818 S Euclid Ave
St Louis, MO 63110-1594
Tel: 314-652-3200

St Joseph's Institute for the Deaf
1483 82nd St
St Louis, MO
Tel: 314-993-1507

Nebraska

Omaha Hearing School for Children, Inc
Karen Glover Rossi
1110 N 66th St
Omaha, NE 68132
Tel: 402-558-1546

Nebraska Commission for the Hearing Impaired
4600 Valley Rd
Lincoln, NE 68510
Tel: 402-471-3593 (voice/TDD)

Boys Town National Research Hospital
555 N 30th St
Omaha, NE 68131
Tel: 402-498-6511 (voice)
402-498-6521 (TDD)

Nevada

Foundation in Auditory Learning
Mary Guski
4353 El Carnal Way
Las Vegas, NV 89121

University of Nevada Dept of Speech Pathology & Audiology
108 Mackay Science Building
Reno, NV 89557
Tel: 702-784-4887

New Hampshire

Alexander Graham Bell Association for the Deaf
Children's Rights Coordinator
Trix Officer
26 Occom Ridge Rd
Hanover, NH 03755
Tel: 603-643-2040

New Hampshire Education Services for the Hearing Impaired
17 S Fruit St
Concord, NH 03301
Tel: 603-225-7073 (voice/TDD)

New Jersey

Alexander Graham Bell Association for the Deaf
Children's Rights Coordinator
Joann Lynch
20 Niles Ave
Middletown, NJ 07748
Tel: 201-671-1619

Summit Speech School for the Hearing Impaired Child
Claire Kantor
34 Upper Overlook Rd
Summit, NJ 07901
Tel: 201-277-3353

Laura Houck Welzer
58 Brooktree Rd
East Windsor, NJ 08520
Tel: 609-443-6782

Deaf Contact "609"
1050 N Kings Hwy
Cherry Hill, NJ 08034
Tel: 609-667-3000 ext 428
609-667-2900 (voice/TDD)

Jewish Deaf and Hearing Impaired Council
199 Scoles Ave
Clifton, NJ 07012
Tel: 201-779-2980 (voice)
201-779-2984 (TDD)

New York

Alexander Graham Bell Association for the Deaf
Robbie O'Hara, Chapter President
61 Vine Rd
Larchmont, NY 10538
Tel: 914-834-7816 (home)

Alexander Graham Bell Association for the Deaf
Children's Rights Coordinators
Bruce Goldstein
56 Fairlawn Dr
Eggertsville, NY 14226
Tel: 716-833-1632 (home)
716-856-1344 (work)

Inez Janger
19 Buena Vista Dr
Hastings-on-Hudson, NY 10706
Tel: 914-478-2415 (home)
516-391-3908 (work)

Catherine McEnroe
1428 Oneida St
Utica, NY 13501

Catholic Charities Bi-County Center Services for the Deaf
143 Schleigel Blvd
Amityville, NY 11801
Tel: 516-842-1400 (voice)
516-842-1540 (TDD)

Southern Tier Independence Center
Marie Dibble, Executive Director
232 Clinton St
Binghamton, NY 13905
Tel: 607-797-1110

Deafness Services, Catholic Charities
191 Joralemon St
Brooklyn, NY 11201
Tel: 718-598-5500 ext 352 (voice)
718-596-0303 (TDD)

**Northeast Communication
Achievement Center**
St Mary's School for the Deaf
2253 Main St
Buffalo, NY 14214
Tel: 716-834-7200 ext 106

**New York League for the
Hard of Hearing**
71 W 23rd St
New York, NY 10010
Tel: 212-741-7650 (voice)
212-255-1932 (TDD)

North Carolina

**Alexander Graham Bell Association
for the Deaf
Children's Rights Coordinator**
Kim Cooper, MA, CCC-SP
Speech/Language Pathologist
New Hanover Memorial Hospital
PO Box 9000
Wilmington, NC 28402
Tel: 919-343-7218

**Asheville Community Service Center
for the Hearing Impaired**
518 Kenilworth Rd, Suite C-5
Asheville, NC 28805
Tel: 704-258-6190 (voice)
704-254-2281 (TDD)

**Charlotte Community Service Center
for the Hearing Impaired**
1926 E Independence Blvd
Charlotte, NC 28205
Tel: 704-334-3481 (voice)
704-334-1687 (TDD)

**Guilford County Communications
Center for the Deaf**
1601 Walker Ave
Greensboro, NC 27403
Tel: 919-274-1461 (voice)
919-275-8878 or
919-883-2912 (TDD)

**North Carolina Council
for the Hearing Impaired**
620 N West St
PO Box 26053
Raleigh, NC 27611
Tel: 919-733-3364 (voice)
919-733-5930 (TDD)

Winston-Salem Deafness Center
2701 N Cherry St
Winston-Salem, NC 27105
Tel: 919-724-3621 (voice)
919-724-7805 (TDD)

North Dakota

**Alexander Graham Bell Association
for the Deaf
Children's Rights Coordinator**
Diane MacDonald
Souris Valley Special Services
215 2nd St, SE
Minot, ND 58705

Medical Center Rehabilitation Hospital
1300 S Columbia Rd
Grand Forks, ND 58201
Tel: 701-780-2447

Ohio

**Alexander Graham Bell Association
for the Deaf**
Elizabeth W. Williams, Chapter President
1572 Rombach Ave
East US 22 & SR 3
Wilmington, OH 45177
Tel: 513-382-4012 (TDD)
513-382-2396 (1st/3rd Tues/Wed)

**Alexander Graham Bell Association
for the Deaf
Children's Rights Coordinators**
Marion Boss, PhD
University of Toledo
Toledo, OH 43606
Tel: 419-472-0099 (home)
419-537-2839 (work)

Sandy Benson
5225 Denise Dr
Dayton, OH 45429

Scott Gordon
587 Crescent Rd
Mansfield, OH 44907
Tel: 419-756-4137 (home)
419-525-6347 (work)

173

Community Services for the Deaf
212 E Exchange St
Akron, OH 44313
Tel: 216-376-9494
 216-376-9351 (TDD)

Cincinnati Speech and Hearing Center
3021 Vernon Pl
Cincinnati, OH 45219
Tel: 513-221-0527 (voice)
 513-221-3300 (TDD)

Community Center for the Deaf
854 W Town St
Columbus, OH 43222
Tel: 614-228-3323 (voice/TDD)

A.C.H.I.C.
Connie Might
1311 Harpster Ave
Akron, OH 44314

Youngstown Hearing and Speech Center
6505 Market St
Youngstown, OH 44512
Tel: 216-726-8855 (voice)
 216-726-8391 (TDD)

Oklahoma

Alexander Graham Bell Association for the Deaf
Children's Rights Coordinator
Cynthia Lindauer
1608 Andover Ct
Oklahoma City, OK 73120
Tel: 405-840-0710 (home)
 405-232-4286 (work)

Oregon

Tucker-Maxon Oral School
Patrick Stone, Director
2860 SE Holgate Blvd
Portland, OR 97202
Tel: 503-235-6551

Regional Resource Center on Deafness
Western Oregon State College
John Freeburg, MS, Director
345 N Monmouth Ave
Monmouth, OR 97361
Tel: 503-838-1220 (voice)
 503-838-5151 (TDD)

Pennsylvania

Alexander Graham Bell Association for the Deaf
Jean Comforo, Chapter President
616 N Lemon St
Media, PA 19063
Tel: 215-565-6964 (voice/TDD)
 215-565-4585 (home)

Alexander Graham Bell Association for the Deaf
Children's Rights Coordinators
Linda L. Abrams
562 Rutter Ave
Kingston, PA 18704
Tel: 717-287-1733

Judith Sexton
Archbishop Ryan Memorial Institute for the Deaf
3509 Spring Garden St
Philadelphia, PA 19104
Tel: 215-667-0654 (home)
 215-387-1711 (work)

Archbishop Ryan Memorial Institute for the Deaf
Sister Mary Therese Toole, SSJ
3509 Spring Garden St
Philadelphia, PA 19104
Tel: 215-387-1711

DePaul Institute
Sr M. Philomena Mannion
Castlegate Ave
Pittsburgh, PA 15226
Tel: 412-561-4848

Lehigh-Northampton Counseling Services for the Deaf, Inc
3028 Liberty St
Allentown, PA 18104
Tel: 215-432-9118 (voice)
 215-435-6123 (TDD)

Bloomsburg University
Dept of Community Disabilities and Special Education
Bloomsburg, PA 17815
Tel: 717-389-4436 (voice/TDD)

Lutheran Social Services, Deaf Center Services
1050 Pennsylvania Ave
York, PA 17404
Tel: 717-848-6238 (voice)
 717-848-6765 (TDD)

Westmoreland County Deaf Services
110 E Otterman St
Greensburg, PA 15601
Tel: 412-832-7600 (voice/TDD)

Berks County Association for the Hearing Impaired
M. Danowski
223 N 6th St
Reading, PA 19601

Center on Deafness
Western Pennsylvania School
300 E Swissvale Ave
Pittsburgh, PA 15218

Pittsburgh Hearing, Speech & Deaf Services
1945 5th Ave
Pittsburgh, PA 15219
Tel: 412-281-1375 (voice/TDD)

South Dakota

Alexander Graham Bell Association for the Deaf
Children's Rights Coordinator
Carol Trebilcock
810 N Main
Aberdeen, SD 57401
Tel: 605-225-6681

Communication Services for the Deaf
421 N Lewis
Sioux Falls, SD 57103
Tel: 605-339-6718 (voice/TDD)

Tennessee

Alexander Graham Bell Association for the Deaf
Children's Rights Coordinators
Mary Trabue Fitzgerald
PO Box 150311
Nashville, TN 37215
Tel: 615-385-2785 (home)
    615-292-4741 (work)

Al Stults
1101 Albany Rd
Knoxville, TN 37923
Tel: 615-691-2116 (home)
    615-482-5302 (work)

Memphis Oral School for the Deaf
Joan H. Ward
711 Jefferson Ave
Memphis, TN 38105
Tel: 901-577-8490

Services for the Deaf
317 Oak St, Suite 316
Chattanooga, TN 37412
Tel: 615-755-2850 (voice)
    615-755-2859 (TDD)

University of Tennessee Language and Communication Program
711 Jefferson Ave
Memphis, TN 38105
Tel: 901-528-6511

Clover Bottom Developmental Center Speech and Hearing Department
275 Stewarts Ferry Pike
Nashville, TN 37214
Tel: 615-889-9247 ext 4506 or 4675

League for the Hearing Impaired, Inc
1810 Edgehill Ave
Nashville, TN 37212
Tel: 615-320-7347 (voice)
    615-329-9271 (TDD)

Texas

Alexander Graham Bell Association for the Deaf
Helen Golf, Chapter President
14007 Red Clover
San Antonio, TX 78231
Tel: 512-492-3921

Alexander Graham Bell Association for the Deaf
Children's Rights Coordinators
Nancy Arias
221 Meadowbrook
San Antonio, TX 78232
Tel: 512-490-3903 (home)
    512-824-0579 (work)

Tammy Chambers
14640 Sweetwater Creek
Corpus Christi, TX 78410
Tel: 512-387-1271

Marilyn Williams
2609 Douglas Dr
Amarillo, TX 79110
Tel: 806-352-4124 (home)

Mary Woodley
5302 75th St, Apt 1104
Lubbock, TX 79424
Tel: 806-798-2625

Dinah Zaleski
2345 Watts Rd
Houston, TX 77030
Tel: 713-664-9920

Houston School for Deaf Children
Sheryl Jorgensen
3636 W Dallas
Houston, TX 77019
Tel: 713-523-3633

Sunshine Cottage for Deaf Children
Dr Wallace Bruce, Director
103 Tuleta Dr
San Antonio, TX 78212
Tel: 512-824-0579

Texas Commission for the Deaf
510 S Congress
Austin, TX 78704
Tel: 512-469-9891 (voice/TDD)

Southeast Texas Council
for the Hearing Impaired
PO Box 1748
Beaumont, TX 77704
Tel: 409-833-6679 (voice)
409-833-6689 (TDD)

Corpus Christi Area Council
for the Deaf
5151 McArdle
Corpus Christi, TX 78411
Tel: 512-993-1154 (voice/TDD)

El Paso Center of the Deaf, Inc
1005 E Yandell
El Paso, TX 79902
Tel: 915-544-6032 (voice/TDD)

Deaf Council of Greater Houston
6910 Fannin, Suite 204
Houston, TX 77030
Tel: 713-796-0520 (voice)
713-796-2416 (TDD)

San Antonio Council for the Deaf
2803 E Commerce
San Antonio, TX 78203
Tel: 512-223-9200 (voice/TDD)

Texoma Council for the Deaf
800 N Travis
Sherman, TX 75090
Tel: 214-892-6531 (voice/TDD)

Utah

Alexander Graham Bell Association
for the Deaf
Parent Section
Thai Williams
426 S 10th E, #607
Salt Lake City, UT 84102
Tel: 801-298-4821

Vermont

Alexander Graham Bell Association
for the Deaf
Children's Rights Coordinator
Wendy Sommer
9 North St
Brattleboro, VT 05301
Tel: 802-257-5549

Virginia

Alexander Graham Bell Association
for the Deaf
Mary Gleason, Chapter President
9601 Renton Dr
Burke, VA 22015
Tel: 703-250-5689

Alexander Graham Bell Association
for the Deaf
Children's Rights Coordinators
Pratibha Srinivasan
Rte 3, Box 1002
Blacksburg, VA 24060
Tel: 703-552-0083 (work)
703-951-4746 (home)

Carleen Wheeler
8100 Guinevere Dr
Annandale, VA 22003
Tel: 703-573-7139

Virginia Department for the Deaf
and Hard of Hearing
James Monroe Building, 7th Floor
1001 N 14th St
Richmond, VA 23219-3678
Tel: 804-225-2570
800-552-7917 (in VA) (voice/TDD)

Washington

Alexander Graham Bell Association
for the Deaf
Carol Randall, Chapter President
12500 Riviera Place NE
Seattle, WA 98125
Tel: 206-364-7013

Alexander Graham Bell Association
for the Deaf
Children's Rights Coordinator
Star Leonard-Fleckman
5041 Ivanhoe Place, NE
Seattle, WA 98105
Tel: 206-525-7256

Early Childhood
Home Instruction Program
EEU WJ-10, University of Washington
Seattle, WA 98195
Tel: 206-543-4011

Hearing, Speech and
Deafness Center
1620 18th Ave
Seattle, WA 98122
Tel: 206-323-5770

West Virginia

Alexander Graham Bell Association for the Deaf
Children's Rights Coordinator
Deborah S. Traylor
65 Derby Lane
Huntington, WV 25705
Tel: 304-525-9380 (home)

Alexander Graham Bell Association for the Deaf
Parent Section
Carrie S. Lambert
1406 Greenbriar St, Apt A
Charleston, WV 25311
Tel: 304-342-8329

Deaf CONTACT
Quarrier & Morris Sts
Charleston, WV 25301
Tel: 304-346-0826 (voice)
 304-346-0828 (TDD)

Wisconsin

Alexander Graham Bell Association for the Deaf
Children's Rights Coordinator
Anna Rentmeester, RN, MSN
2207 Mt View Blvd
Wausau, WI 54401
Tel: 715-848-2638 (home)
 715-847-5888 (work)

Office for Hearing Impaired
718 W Clairemont Ave
Eau Claire, WI 54701
Tel: 713-836-2062 (voice/TDD)

Office for the Hearing Impaired
One W Wilson St, Room 412
PO Box 7851
Madison, WI 53707
Tel: 608-266-8081 (voice)
 608-266-8083 (TDD)

Canada

Alexander Graham Bell Association for the Deaf
Lucia Harold, Chapter President
83 Sunset Dr
Regina, Saskatchewan
Canada S4S 2R6

Alexander Graham Bell Association for the Deaf
Children's Rights Coordinator
Ann Jexewski
PO Box 1438
26 Clay St
Almonte, Ontario
Canada K0A 1A0
Tel: 613-256-1850

Vancouver Oral Centre for Deaf Children, Inc
Hilda Gregory
4824 Commercial St
Vancouver, British Columbia
Canada V5N 4H1
Tel: 604-874-0255

Montreal Oral School for the Deaf, Inc
Agnes H. Phillips, PhD, Principal
5851 Upper Lachine Rd
Montreal, Quebec
Canada H4A 2B7
Tel: 514-488-4946

PREVIOUSLY PUBLISHED ROSS CONFERENCE AND ROUNDTABLE REPORTS

Reports of Ross Conferences on Pediatric Research

Title	Date of Publication
1. Megaloblastic Anemia	8/51
2. Retrolental Fibroplasia	11/51
3. Carbohydrate Metabolism	4/52
4. Calcium and Phosphorus Metabolism	10/52
5. Pulmonary Hyaline Membranes	2/53
6. Potassium Metabolism	5/53
7. Erythroblastosis Fetalis	4/54
8. Renal Function in Infants and Children	2/54
9. Immunity and Hypersensitivity Relationship to Disease in Man	3/55
10. Vitamin B_6 in Human Nutrition	6/54
11. Fat Metabolism	10/54
12. Diabetes Mellitus in Infants and Children	2/55
13. Adrenal Function in Infants and Children	6/55
14. Congenital Heart Disease	12/55
15. Respiratory Problems in the Premature Infant	10/55
16. Retrolental Fibroplasia—Role of Oxygen	1/56
17. Growth and Development of Dental and Skeletal Tissue—Clinical and Biological Aspects	2/56
18. Fibrocystic Disease of the Pancreas	4/56
19. Metabolism and Function of Iron	6/56
20. Thyroid and Iodine Metabolism	2/57
21. Psychological Aspects in the Care of Infants and Children	11/56
22. Mesenchymal Diseases in Childhood	4/57
23. Etiologic Factors in Mental Retardation	8/57
24. Psychological Implications of Current Pediatric Practice	11/57
25. Consciousness and the Chemical Environment of the Brain	2/58
26. Physical and Behavioral Growth	6/58
27. The Nonoperative Aspects of Pediatric Surgery	10/58
28. The Child at Law	12/58
29. Immunity and Resistance to Infection in Early Infancy	3/59
30. Amino Acid and Protein Metabolism	4/59
31. Adaptation to Extrauterine Life	7/59
32. Disturbances of Cellular Metabolism in Infancy	10/59
33. Perspectives in Pediatric Virology	1/60
34. Current Concepts in Leukemia	9/60
35. Endocrine Dysfunction and Infertility	1/61
36. Careers in Pediatrics	10/60
37. Normal and Abnormal Respiration in Children	3/61
38. The Normal Cell and Its Response to Allergic Stimuli	10/61
39. Circadian Systems	12/61
40. Mechanisms of Regulation of Growth	6/62
41. Perinatal Pharmacology	10/62
Supplement No. 1	
Techniques of Exchange Transfusion	12/62

42. Recent Advances in Degenerative Diseases of the Central Nervous System in Infants and Children	2/63
43. Medical Responsibilities for the Displaced Child	4/63
44. Psychosomatic Aspects of Gastrointestinal Illness in Childhood	9/63
45. Clinical Use of Radioisotopes in Pediatrics	11/63

Supplement No. 2

Thermoregulation of the Newly Born	4/64
46. Physical Diagnosis of the Newly Born	5/64
47. International Child Health	9/64
48. Aplastic Anemia	3/65
49. Problems in Neonatal Surgery	7/65
50. Macromolecular Aspects of Protein Absorption and Excretion in the Mammalian Intestine	1/65
51. Juvenile Diabetes Mellitus	6/65
52. Fetal Hemoglobin	6/66
53. Intrauterine Transfusion and Erythroblastosis Fetalis	9/66
54. Human Pituitary Growth Hormone	10/66
55. Overwhelming Bacterial Infections in Childhood	12/66
56. Assessing the Effectiveness of Child Health Services	10/67
57. Brain Damage in the Fetus and Newborn From Hypoxia or Asphyxia	11/67
58. Problems of Drug Evaluation in Infants and Children	10/68
59. Problems of Neonatal Intensive Care Units	3/69
60. Problems of Nutrition in the Perinatal Period	5/70
61. Learning Disorders in Children	1/71
62. Iron Nutrition in Infancy	11/70
63. A Search for a Better Way: The Future of Child Health Services	1/72
64. Slow Virus Infections	10/73
65. Ethical Dilemmas in Current Obstetric and Newborn Care	10/73
66. Regionalization of Perinatal Care	10/74
67. The Care of Children With Chronic Illnesses	3/75
68. Necrotizing Enterocolitis in the Newborn Infant	8/75
69. Iatrogenic Problems in Neonatal Intensive Care	4/76
70. Lung Maturation and the Prevention of Hyaline Membrane Disease	2/77
71. Apnea of Prematurity	4/77
72. Gastrointestinal Development and Neonatal Nutrition	4/77
73. The Roles of Family Practice, Internal Medicine, Obstetrics and Gynecology and Pediatrics in Providing Primary Care	6/77
74. Etiology, Pathophysiology, and Treatment of Acute Gastroenteritis	8/78
75. The Ductus Arteriosus	11/78
76. Gastroesophageal Reflux	5/79
77. Neonatal Neurological Assessment and Outcome	3/80
78. Obstetrical Decisions and Neonatal Outcome	5/81
79. Feeding the Neonate Weighing Less Than 1500 Grams—Nutrition and Beyond	2/81
80. Arthritis in Childhood	5/81
81. The Mucosal Immune System in Health and Disease	6/81
82. Iron Nutrition Revisited—Infancy, Childhood, Adolescence	8/81
83. Cardiovascular Sequelae of Asphyxia in the Newborn	5/82
84. Chemical and Radiation Hazards to Children	11/82
85. Hyperbilirubinemia in the Newborn	9/83
86. Management of Pharyngitis in an Era of Declining Rheumatic Fever	1/84

87. Neonatal Cholestasis: Causes, Syndromes, Therapies	11/84
88. Children's Blood Pressure	4/85
89. Somatomedins and Other Peptide Growth Factors: Relevance to Pediatrics	10/85
90. Bronchopulmonary Dysplasia and Related Chronic Respiratory Disorders	3/86
91. The Breastfed Infant: A Model for Performance	10/86
92. Frontiers in Genetic Medicine	9/87
93. Infant of the Diabetic Mother	11/87
94. Enteral Feeding: Scientific Basis and Clinical Applications	5/88
95. Prevention of Adult Atherosclerosis During Childhood	8/88
96. Surfactant Treatment of Lung Diseases	11/88
97. Emergency Medical Services for Children	5/89
98. Body Composition Measurements in Infants and Children	9/89
99. The Micropremie: The Next Frontier	4/90
100. The Term Newborn Infant: A Current Look	5/91
101. Developmental Mechanisms of Disease in the Newborn	12/91

Reports of Ross Roundtables
on Critical Approaches to Common Pediatric Problems

Title	*Date of Publication*
1. Urinary Tract Infections in Childhood	12/69
2. Obesity in Pediatric Practice	2/71
3. Common Orthopedic Conditions in Childhood	7/73
4. A Problem-Oriented Approach to Upper Respiratory Tract Conditions in Childhood	9/74
5. Hypersensitivity Problems in Pediatric Practice	9/75
6. Contemporary Management of Emergency Problems in Pediatrics: The Critical First Hours	10/76
7. Adolescent Gynecology	3/77
8. Child Advocacy and Pediatrics	2/78
9. School-Related Health Care	4/79
10. Sports Medicine for Children and Youth	10/79
11. Counseling the Mother on Breast-Feeding	4/80
12. Preventing Childhood Injuries	1/82
13. Diagnosis and Management of Acute Diarrhea	8/82
14. Adolescent Substance Abuse	7/83
15. The Adolescent Family	6/84
16. Daycare	7/85
17. Well-Child Care	7/86
18. Medical-Legal Issues in Pediatrics	8/87
19. The Febrile Infant and Occult Bacteremia	8/88
20. Pediatric AIDS	12/89
21. Pediatric Asthma	8/90
22. Child Sexual Abuse	9/91
23. Children and Violence	In preparation

NOTE: These publications may be available in medical school and pediatric department libraries.